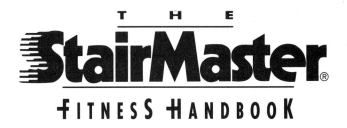

FITNESS HANDBOOK

A User's Guide
To Exercise Testing
And Prescription

foreword by

BRUNO BALKE, MD, PHD

James A. Peterson, Ph.D.   *Cedric X. Bryant, Ph.D.*

● ●

Published by Masters Press (a subsidiary of Howard W. Sams)
2647 Waterfront Pkwy E. Dr., Suite 300, Indianapolis, IN 46214

First edition.

Library of Congress Catalog-in-Publication Data

The StairMaster fitness handbook/edited by James A. Peterson
    and Cedric X. Bryant.
        p.   cm.
        Includes bibliographical references.
        ISBN 0-940279-44-4: $12.95
        1. Exercise 2. Physical fitness. 3. Aerobic exercise.
I. Peterson, James A., 1943- . II. Bryant, Cedric X., 1960 - .
RA781.S697   1992   92-1616
613.7'1--dc20   CIP

Book design: Laura Griswold
Cover design: Agency X

FOREWORD

Life is action—movement affects and forms total life! Insufficient physical challenges in our civilization have been shown to result in functional degeneration, as evidenced by the enormous number of heart and vascular diseases in countries with the highest standards of living.

Shortly after the end of the last great war, it was not unusual for any pursuit of voluntary physical exercise to be ridiculed. As a consequence, "physical fitness" in American children and adults was at an undesirably low level, as shown by several pertinent studies.

With the founding of the American College of Sports Medicine in 1954, a significant change in the lethargic behavior and attitudes of the general population was initiated. Medical doctors and exercise physiologists undertook numerous scientific investigations into the effects of inactivity, as well as of physical training on a regular basis, on health and fitness. The leadership provided by the spoken words, the writings and the personal examples of these individuals served as a major stimulus for the growing number of exercise enthusiasts in this country.

Since "fads" come and go, many individuals were concerned that this new level of active participation in sports and recreational activities might be a termporary phenomenon. Such an undesirable consequence, however, seems most unlikely to occur since too many men and women have experienced the many benefits that accrue in their own lives as a consequence of individual adherence to any of the many positive forms of physical activity.

Forty years ago, the author of this foreword was engaged in teaching a theoretical, as well as practical, course concerned with the physiological reactions and functional adaptations to regularly performed "aerobic" exercise. The "students" were medical officers at the United States Air Force School of Aerospace Medicine in San Antonio, Texas. One of the officers who participated in the training program experienced personal changes in his own body attendant to a more healthy life style. Subsequently, he declared his intention to stir up the mood of the American population to become more active. And indeed, he did just that by coining the term "AEROBICS," as a replacement for the somewhat dreadful words "physical education" and "calisthenics." This new term caught on quickly. As a result, many aerobic types of physical activity became not only more popular, but even "fashionable."

Since that time millions of people have joined the fitness "band wagon." The enthusiasm and efforts of these individuals have contributed to the awareness concerning the innumerable benefits that await those who engage in a sound exercise program. For those of you who are already exercise "converts," *The StairMaster® Fitness Handbook* was written to help preserve your discipline and desire to maintain a level of optimal performance capacity into "old age." For those of you who have been advised to change to a healthier life style or have decided on your own for whatever reasons to become more physically active, this book was designed to provide the basic understanding regarding the "why" and "how" you can exercise reasonably and regularly.

The reader should keep in mind that not all of the chapters are written for everyone. Some of the chapters may only have a unique appeal to health professionals who want to reinforce their knowledge or understanding of the scientific basis of matters about which they are going to "preach." Other chapters, or parts of them, may be more important initially to those individuals who are just on the verge of embarking on a new adventure of initiating a sound exercise program.

In a book with contributions by several authors with similar interests, many repetitions were unavoidable. Such repetitions, however, can only serve to reinforce certain important issues.

StairMaster Sports/Medical Products, Inc. should be commended for making *The StairMaster® Fitness Handbook* available, not only to its customers, but also to anyone who is interested in the health benefits of a sound exercise program— regardless of the type of equipment used.

Bruno Balke, M.D., Ph.D.

● ●

"We doctors can now state from our experience with people, both sick and well, and from a growing series of scientific researches that 'keeping fit' does pay richly in dividends of health and longevity."

Paul Dudley White, M.D.

CONTRIBUTORS

Victor Ben-Ezra, Ph.D.
Associate Professor
Dept. of Kinesiology
Texas Woman's University
Denton, Texas

Donald Bergey, M.A.
Exercise Coordinator
Cardiac Rehabilitation Program
Dept. of Medicine, Health
and Sport Science
Wake Forest University
Winston-Salem, North Carolina

Dennis Colacino, Ph.D.
Professor
New York Medical College
Valhalla, New York

M. Elaine Cress, Ph.D.
Senior Research Fellow
Dept. of Medicine
Division of Gerontology
and Geriatric Medicine
University of Washington
Seattle, Washington

Debra J. Crews, Ph.D.
Assistant Professor
Dept. of Exercise and Sport Science
University of North Carolina
at Greensboro
Greensboro, North Carolina

Todd Crowder, Ph.D.
Director of Sports Medicine
United States Military Academy
Dept. of Physical Education
West Point, New York

Karol Fink, B.S.
Nutritional Sciences Program
University of Washington
Seattle, Washington

B. Don Franks, Ph.D.
Professor and Chair
Dept. of Kinesiology
Louisiana State University
Baton Rouge, Louisiana

Larry W. Gibbons, M.D.
Medical Director
The Cooper Clinic
Dallas, Texas

James E. Graves, Ph.D.
Research Associate
Center for Exercise Science
University of Florida
Gainesville, Florida

Gary Gray, P.T.
Director
Gary Gray Physical Therapy
Adrian, Michigan

Elizabeth Hart M.A.
Dept. of Exercise and Sport Science
University of North Carolina
at Greensboro
Greensboro, North Carolina

David L. Herbert, Esq.
Senior Partner
Herbert, Benson & Scott,
Attorneys at Law
Canton, Ohio

William G. Herbert, Ph.D.
Professor and Director
Laboratory for Exercise, Sport and
Work Physiology
Virginia Polytechnic Institute
Blacksburg, Virginia

James L. Hodgson, Ph.D.
Associate Professor of Applied
Physiology
Noll Human Performance Laboratory
Pennsylvania State University
University Park, Pennsylvania

George J. Holland, Ph.D.
Professor and Co-Director
Exercise Physiology Laboratory
California State University,
Northridge
Northridge, California

W. Larry Kenney, Ph.D.
Associate Professor of Applied
Physiology
Noll Human Performance Laboratory
Pennsylvania State University
University Park, Pennsylvania

Steven F. Loy, Ph.D.
Associate Professor and Co-Director
Exercise Physiology Laboratory
California State University
Northridge, California

W. Channing Nicholas, M.D.
General Practitioner/Assoc. Professor
of Applied Physiol. Professor
Noll Human Performance Laboratory
Pennsylvania State University
University Park, Pennsylvania

Michael L. Pollock, Ph.D.
Director
Center for Exercise Science
University of Florida
Gainesville, Florida

Paul M. Ribisl, Ph.D.
Director
Cardiac Rehabilitation Program
Dept. of Medicine, Health,
and Sport Science
Wake Forest University
Winston-Salem, North Carolina

James S. Skinner, Ph.D.
Professor
Dept. of Exercise Science and
Physical Education
Arizona State University
Tempe, Arizona

Neil Sol, Ph.D.
General Manager
The Houstonian Club
Houston, Texas

Karl G. Stoedefalke, Ph.D.
Professor
Dept. of Exercise and Sport Science
Pennsylvania State University
University Park, Pennsylvania

Gerald D. Thompson, M.S.
Dept. of Kinesiology
Louisiana State University
Baton Rouge, Louisiana

Wayne L. Westcott, Ph.D.
Fitness Director
South Shore YMCA
Quincy, Massachusetts

Cary Wing, M.A.
Director
HeartHealth Cardiac Rehabilitation, Inc.
Poughkeepsie, New York

Bonnie Worthington-Roberts, Ph.D.
Professor and Director
Nutritional Sciences Program
University of Washington
Seattle, Washington

LIST OF TABLES

List Of Figures

CONTENTS

If you should have any questions pertaining to the information presented in this book, please contact:

StairMaster Sports/Medical Products, Inc.
Attn.: Department of Sports Medicine
12421 Willows Road NE, Ste 100
Kirkland, WA 98034

PROLOGUE:

•••••••••••••••••••••••••••••••••••

ABOUT THIS BOOK

*T*he *StairMaster® Fitness Handbook* is an extension of the corporate philosophy of StairMaster® Sports/Medical Products, Inc. to lend support to projects that are designed to enable individuals to become more knowledgeable about what constitutes "sensible exercise." Previous endeavors that reflect this corporate commitment to disseminate information relating to the benefits and parameters of sensible exercise include the sponsorship of several projects conducted by the American College of Sports Medicine and the development of one of the most extensive programs of independently conducted, applied research in the therapeutic and fitness equipment industry.

Collectively, the *StairMaster® Fitness Handbook* features the writings of 28 individuals whose contributions enabled this book to become a reality. The contributors' thorough mastery of their subject matter served as the basis for providing a comprehensive overview of several critical issues relating to exercise, including why you should exercise, *what* physiological responses occur as the result of exercising, and *what* type of exercise prescriptions produce optimal results. Every attempt was made to make the information included in this book as user-friendly as possible.

As you read the *StairMaster® Fitness Handbook,* you should keep in mind that becoming knowledgeable about exercise is only one of many essential ingredients in your personal recipe for sensible exercise. If you want to make your "exercise experience" as productive and enjoyable as possible, you need to take several steps. Undoubtedly, the most critical step is that you make an unwavering commitment to exercise on a regular basis. For most individuals, that commitment will be based—at least in part—on an understanding of the fact that regular exercise participation makes sense for almost everyone and that exercise truly has medicinal properties. Hopefully, *The StairMaster® Fitness Handbook* will serve to facilitate that understanding and, as a result, strengthen your resolve to exercise in a safe and appropriate manner.

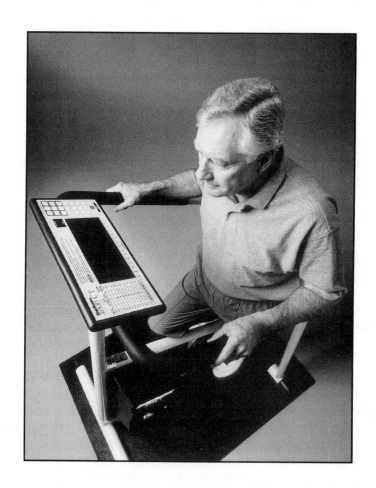

CHAPTER 1

. . . .

EXERCISE IS MEDICINE

by

Larry Gibbons, M.D.
and
Karl Stoedefalke, Ph.D.

• • •

C. Everett Koop, during his tenure as the Surgeon General of the United States, had one of his researchers add up all of the people known to be suffering from the various major diseases reported by the National Center for Health Statistics. Somewhat astonishingly, the researcher found that the total exceeded the entire population of the United States. The major point to be inferred from this fact is that health—specifically the lack of health—is perhaps the most critical issue currently facing the American society.

Attempts to identify the factors which have been major contributors to this virtual epidemic of medical problems have produced a litany of probable reasons why such a large number of individuals are so apparently unhealthy . . . poor eating habits, a sedentary lifestyle, stress, poor health habits (i.e., smoking), ad infinitum. At the same time, a number of studies have been undertaken to identify what—if anything—can be done to diminish either the number or the severity of medical problems affecting the public. These studies have provided considerable evidence that exercise has substantial medicinal benefits for individuals of all ages.

Two of the most widely publicized efforts to investigate the possible relationship between exercise and disease were longitudinal studies, each of which involved more than 10,000 subjects. Several years ago, in a renowned study of 17,000 Harvard graduates, Ralph Paffenbarger, M.D., found that men who expended approximately 300 calories a day—the equivalent of walking briskly for 45 minutes—reduced their death rates from all causes by an extraordinary 28% and lived an average of more than two years longer than their sedentary former classmates. A more recent study conducted by Steven Blair, P.E.D., of the Institute of Aerobics Research in Dallas documented the fact that a relatively modest amount of exercise has a significant effect on the mortality rate of both men and women. The higher the fitness level, the lower the death rate (after the data was adjusted for age differences between subjects in this eight-year investigation of 13,344 individuals). An analysis of the extensive data yielded by both studies suggests one inescapable conclusion—*EXERCISE IS MEDICINE*.

REDUCING YOUR RISK FOR CAD

The number one cause of death of men and women in the United States is coronary artery disease (CAD). In 1991 alone more than 800,000 deaths could be directly attributed to CAD. Unfortunately, even though CAD has been found to begin relatively early in life (sometimes as early as the teenage years for males), the symptoms of this horrific condition do not occur until the disease is far advanced in an individual. Almost twenty-five percent of the individuals with CAD suffer a fatal heart attack as their initial symptom of this disease. Given the nature of CAD, "prevention" is, without question, the most appropriate approach to this pandemic medical problem.

Of all the major interventive steps that an individual can take to help prevent the onset of CAD—change of lifestyle, cessation of cigarette smoking, weight control, and eating a nutritionally balanced diet—exercise has generally been found to be the cornerstone of an effort that combines several interventions. Exercise has been shown to have a substantial effect on the most critical (and modifiable) risk factors for CAD.

Exercise helps to prevent CAD by affecting an individual's blood lipid level in a positive way. For example, regular exercise has been found to raise high density lipoprotein (HDL—the "good" type) cholesterol levels. HDL cholesterol is more important than low density lipoprotein (LDL—the "bad" type) cholesterol apparently because of its ability to help protect against CAD by its efforts to collect cholesterol in the body's blood system and help dispose of it safely in the liver. By transferring cholesterol to the liver, HDL helps prevent the accumulation of lipids on walls of the arteries (a process commonly referred to as atherosclerosis). By facilitating the formation of HDL and helping to slow the eventual breakdown of HDL, exercise enables individuals to have higher levels of this cardioprotective lipoprotein.

Exercise also helps to prevent CAD by enabling individuals to keep their blood pressure level under control. High blood pressure (a condition commonly referred to as hypertension) is a state in which the blood pressure is chronically elevated above optimal levels. Regular exercise has been found to lower both systolic and diastolic blood pressure. The average lowering of blood pressure with exercise has been shown to be approximately 10 mm Hg and 8 mm Hg for systolic and diastolic blood pressure, respectively. Recent studies show that a 7-mm Hg reduction in diastolic blood pressure, for example, will reduce the incidence of CAD by approximately 29% and the incidence of stroke by 46%. Not surprisingly, individuals who already suffer from high blood pressure can significantly lower their mortality risk by exercising on a regular basis.

Exercise has also been shown to help prevent CAD by aiding some people (not all) in their attempts to quit smoking. Some evidence exists to suggest that an individual's craving for cigarettes is reduced with exercise participation. Other studies have found that many individuals who had previously smoked voluntarily gave up this habit once they became involved in a program of regular physical activity. Unfortunately, the addictive qualities of nicotine (nicotine is a drug which is six to eight times more addictive than alcohol) override, in many instances, a smoker's capacity to adequately consider the beneficial consequences of exercise. At the present time, statistics indicate that more than 50 million Americans still smoke.

Exercise has also been found to play a major role in lowering body fat. Obesity is a significant risk factor for CAD. Individuals who are "over-fat" have a substantially higher risk of heart disease—particularly when the body fat is accumulated around their waists. Regular exercise helps to improve body composition in primarily two ways. One way is by increasing caloric expenditure, and thereby creating a caloric deficit. If a previously sedentary individual walks two miles a day at a speed of 4 mph, five days a week, that person can expect to lose about 9.5 to 11.0 pounds over a one-year period of time—provided caloric intake remains stable.* The other way in which exercise helps to improve body composition is by ensuring that the majority of weight loss is from fat rather than lean body tissue. In addition to its positive effects on body composition, exercise also helps to counteract several of the negative consequences of being over-fat, such as high blood pressure, glucose intolerance, a low level of HDL cholesterol in the blood, and low self-esteem.

MORE EXERCISE, LESS DRUGS

In recent years, many health experts have concluded that medical science has (for many chronic health problems) achieved about as much as can be expected in the battle against sickness and death. Furthermore, based upon an increasing amount of evidence, many experts have surmised that additional expenditures for health care cannot and will not produce the financial benefits that could be achieved if every American adopted better health practices—particularly a physically active lifestyle. In the past three decades, several major epidemiological studies have demonstrated that regular physical activity is associated with an improved quality of life and longevity. And yet, several chronic health problems and conditions exist that are still treated solely with conventional medical therapy. For whatever reason, many members of the medical community are unaware of the therapeutic—as opposed to preventative—role that exercise can have in health care.

In numerous instances, exercise can be an extremely effective adjunct treatment modality for individuals suffering from a diverse array of chronic

---

* Authors' note: These calculations are based on individuals of average size —women (60 kg) and men (70 kg).

medical problems. As a result, properly prescribed exercise programs can lower health care costs, not only by reducing the incidence or severity of health problems in many cases, but also when illness does occur by diminishing an individual's reliance on drugs and limited medical resources.

Any listing of the medical problems and health-related conditions that can be at least partially treated and controlled by exercise would be extensive. Among the most significant of these health concerns are the following:

1. **Hypertension** is a condition, as previously stated, in which an individual's resting blood pressure is chronically above optimal levels. An estimated 60 million American adults have high blood pressure. Hypertension adds to the workload of the heart and arteries and contributes to heart failure and arteriosclerosis. Research has shown that low-intensity (50-70% of $\dot{V}O_2$ max) aerobic exercise can lower systolic blood pressure by 5 to 25 mm Hg and diastolic blood pressure by 3 to 15 mm Hg in mild-to-moderate hypertensives. Of the several possible mechanisms by which training could lower resting blood pressure, a decrease in sympathetic nervous system activity has received the most experimental support. A reduction in sympathetic nerve activity could lower one or both of the two principal determinants of blood pressure (mean arterial blood pressure equals the product of cardiac output and total peripheral resistance).

2. **Anxiety and depression** are the two most prevalent of all mental disorders in the United States. During any given six-month period, up to twenty percent of the U.S. population is affected by either or both of these common symptoms of an individual's failure to properly cope with mental or emotional stress. Exercise can have a positive effect on reducing the $22 billion that is expended in direct costs on mental health care in the United States every year. Exercise has been shown to increase the brain's emission of alpha waves—the brain waves associated with a relaxed meditation-like state of mind. Researchers have also speculated that exercise decreases depression by altering the levels of certain neurotransmitters (norepinephrine, dopamine, and serotonin) in the brain. The majority of studies have involved subjects engaging in aerobic forms of exercise. The ability of resistance exercise to relieve anxiety and depression remains to be seen.

3. **Hypercholesterolemia** is a condition in which the amount of cholesterol in your blood is above an optimal level. Approximately one-fourth of all American adults have blood cholesterol levels above 240 mg/dl (mortality rates for coronary heart disease climb steadily when serum cholesterol levels rise above 180 mg/dl. Numerous studies have documented the fact that physically active people have cholesterol profiles consistent with a lower risk of coronary heart disease. Exercise training produces two very positive plasma lipid and lipoprotein changes in the individual suffering from hypercholesterolemia—it lowers the plasma triglyceride

level and raises the high density lipoprotein (HDL—the so-called "good" lipoprotein particle in your blood) level. To date, this training effect has been more consistently demonstrated in males than in females.

4. **Low back pain** is the most costly medical problem in American society for the 30-60 age group. Across all age groups, it has been estimated that more than 30 million Americans are afflicted with this painful malady. Despite its seriousness, a fail-safe treatment for low back pain has yet to be identified. In a number of instances, however, exercise has been found to be an effective means for both preventing and treating low back pain by enabling an individual to restore proper muscular balance (between abdominal and low back muscles) and to achieve proper flexibility (primarily in the iliopsoas, erector spinae, and hamstring muscle groups).

5. **Peripheral vascular occlusive disease (PVOD)** is a major health problem in the United States that affects over 14 million individuals at any given time. Resulting from restricted (reduced) blood flow to (most commonly) the lower extremities due to arterial obstruction, PVOD can be very painful and may lead in some instances to the development of gangrene and eventual amputation. Exercise training has been shown to be effective in controlling PVOD and in improving the physical capabilities of PVOD sufferers. While the exact mechanisms for these positive responses are not precisely known, researchers advance several plausible explanations. The following mechanisms have been most often suggested: an increase in collateral circulation whereby previously "dormant" blood vessels are used to reroute blood around the site of obstruction; reduced blood viscosity allowing for an easier passage of blood through the narrowed vessel; selective redistribution of blood away from inactive muscles in order that exercising muscles receive a greater supply of blood; biomechanical alteration of gait in which walking patterns are changed such that the metabolic demands placed upon the muscles affected by the disease are reduced; greater extraction of oxygen from the blood by the exercising muscles; and improved pain tolerance resulting from repeated pain exposures during training. Whatever the responsible mechanism(s), a leading authority has stated that exercise training is the most successful and cost effective treatment for PVOD.

6. **Osteoporosis** is an age-related disorder that is characterized by a decreased bone mineral content and has been estimated to be responsible for 1.3 million bone fractures per year. Some evidence exists that exercise retards bone mineral loss. Studies have shown that appropriate exercise can even increase bone density. When gravity stress or muscle movement stress is applied to the bone, the pressure produces a desirable adaptive response within the bone. Training-induced improvements in muscle strength and balance may provide an added benefit by preventing the falls that cause a great number of the fractures occurring among the elderly.

7. **Diabetes mellitus** is the name given to a group of disorders (collectively called diabetes) characterized by metabolic abnormalities, of which the most prominent is an improper handling of glucose (sugar) by the body's cells, resulting in elevated blood glucose levels (the hallmark sign of diabetes). Diabetes is a very serious health problem in the United States. It is the cause of approximately 36,000 deaths annually and is a contributing factor in an additional 95,000 deaths. It is also costly. More than $18 billion is spent in the U.S. to treat diabetes each year. The majority of diabetics are classified as either Type I/insulin-dependent (the pancreas doesn't produce sufficient amounts of insulin), or Type II/non-insulin dependent (the body's cells don't respond appropriately to the insulin produced by the pancreas). Exercise has been shown to be a beneficial adjunct therapy for both types (particularly Type II). A clearly demonstrated effect of aerobic forms of exercise is improved glucose uptake by exercising muscle, which can last up to 72 hours following the exercise bout. By exercising on a regular basis, some individuals with Type II diabetes who require medication to control their blood sugar level are able to reduce or eliminate their need for drugs. Finally, exercise improves a diabetic's blood lipid profile and helps control their blood pressure. By raising HDL-C levels, lowering triglyceride levels and blood pressure, exercise helps protect the diabetic's blood vessels from atherosclerosis (fatty deposits in the arteries). It should also be noted that evidence is accumulating which shows that strength training exercise may also enhance the ability of the body's cells to utilize glucose.

One of the most overriding insights that can be acquired from the aforementioned information concerning the documented relationship between regular exercise and the major health concerns is that exercise can provide a terrific R_x for effective health care. "More exercise, less drugs" should be the standard prescription—not the exception—for those individuals interested in achieving and maintaining a healthy lifestyle.

SLOWING DOWN THE AGING CLOCK

A critical question regarding the aging process centers around whether exercise can slow down the irreversible physiologic changes that occur over the course of an individual's lifetime. The answer is unequivocally "yes," although no one can be certain of the precise extent to which exercise can influence the manner in which an individual's bodily systems respond to aging.

Several of the major changes that occur as an individual ages are of substantial importance. Of particular interest is the fact that many of the changes that accompany aging are similar to those associated with a sedentary lifestyle. At the very least, a physically active lifestyle should have a positive impact on the amount of deterioration experienced by the various physiologic systems of the body since physical activity should help to preserve or maintain higher levels of physiologic function.

One of the primary means by which exercise can exert a positive effect on the aging process involves the cardiorespiratory system. Numerous investigative efforts have shown that elderly individuals who exercise maintain a higher proportion of their cardiorespiratory fitness level than those who don't. As evidence of this, even though $\dot{V}O_2$ max declines in everyone as we get older, physically active individuals are able to slow their average rate of decline in $\dot{V}O_2$ max to a level approximately half that of their sedentary counterparts. Other positive physiological responses include an increase in plasma volume, hemoglobin, muscle glycogen, mitochondrial and oxidative enzyme activity, and oxygen pulse (the amount of oxygen delivered to the working muscles per contraction of the heart) and a reduction in both blood lactate concentrations and heart rate at submaximal work rates.

The other major way that exercise impacts the rate and degree of aging is through its effects on the musculoskeletal system. Several recent studies have supported the contention that strength training can have positive effects on the rate of deterioration of the musculoskeletal system typically observed in older persons. The results of these studies indicated that strength did not decrease substantially with age as it often does (for example, individuals typically suffer a 20-30 percent loss in strength by age 65). In fact, many individuals exhibited dramatic increases in strength. Some subjects in these studies also experienced muscle hypertrophy (an increase in muscle size), in contrast to the usual decrease that occurs. These increases in muscle strength and size tend to translate into improved gait, balance, mobility, and, consequently, better functional capabilities and a lower susceptibility for falling. Also, strength training and low-impact weight-bearing aerobic exercises have been shown to produce increases in bone mineral content in elderly adults.

The American Medical Association's Council on Scientific Affairs states unequivocally that exercise can improve the quality of life for the elderly. Limited functional capabilities and "slowing down" are not and should not be viewed as inevitable consequences of attaining a certain age. The available scientific data indicate that much of the decline in function of a physiologic system is dependent upon the degree to which that system is used. In other words, many changes associated with old age are influenced more by lifestyle than by simply the passage of time. Regardless of how old you are, if you eat right and exercise more, you'll live better. A strong argument could be made that an individual's dignity and sense of independence are inexorably intertwined. The cornerstone of both factors is the ability to be able to do things for yourself. Exercise enhances the likelihood that you will have that ability.

FIT TO LIVE

The old adage, "add life to your years, as well as years to your life," has considerable merit. A sound exercise program can contribute to the quality of your life in countless ways. Are the positive consequences which result from exercising worth the effort involved? Without question. Put another way, is the squirt worth the squeeze? Without a doubt. Should you make exercise an integral part of your daily routine? Of course, you should. In many ways, your life depends on it. ❏

BIBLIOGRAPHY •

1.   American College of Sports Medicine. *Guidelines for Exercise Testing and Exercise Prescription.* Philadelphia, PA: Lea & Febiger, 1991.
2.   American College of Sports Medicine. *Resource Manual for Exercise Testing and Exercise Prescription.* Philadelphia, PA: Lea and Febiger, 1988.
3.   Bouchard, C., Shephard, R.J., Stephens, T., et al. (Eds). *Exercise, Fitness, and Health.* Champaign, IL: Human Kinetics Publishers, 1990.
4.   Duncan, J.J., Farr, J.E., Upton, S.J., et al. "The effects of aerobic exercise on plasma catecholamines and blood pressure in patients with mild essential hypertension." *JAMA* 254:2609-2613, 1985.
5.   Eckert, H.M., Montoye, H.J. (Eds). *Exercise and Health.* Champaign, IL: Human Kinetics Publishers, 1984.
6.   Ernst, E. "Physical exercise for peripheral vascular disease—a review." *Vasa* 16:227-231, 1987.
7.   Franklin, B.A., Gordon, S., Timmis, G.C., et al. (Eds). *Exercise in Modern Medicine.* Baltimore, MD: Williams & Wilkins, 1989.
8.   Gordon, N.F., Scott, C.B., Wilkinson, W.J., et al. "Exercise and mild essential hypertension: Recommendations for adults." *Sports Med* 10(6):390-404, 1990.
9.   Hiatt, W.R., Regensteiner, J.G., Hargarten, M.E., et al. "Benefit of exercise conditioning for patients with peripheral arterial disease." *Circulation* 81:602-609, 1990.
10. Horton, E.S. "Role and management of exercise in diabetes mellitus." *Diabetes Care* 11:201-211, 1988.
11. Morgan, W.P., O'Connor, P.J. "Exercise and mental health." *In* Dishman, R.K. (Ed), *Exercise Adherence.* Champaign, IL: Human Kinetics Publishers, 1988.
12. Peterson, J.A., Wheeler, J. *The Goodbye Back Pain Handbook.* Grand Rapids, MI: Masters Press, 1988.
13. Sinaki, M. "Exercise and osteoporosis." *Arch Phys Med Rehabil* 70:220-229, 1989.
14. Tipton, C.M. "Exercise, training and hypertension: An update." *Exerc Sport Sci Rev* 19:447-505, 1991.

CHAPTER 2

• •

GUIDELINES FOR PRE-EXERCISE HEALTH SCREENING

by

Neil Sol, Ph.D.
and
Cary Wing, M.A.

• • •

*P*rior to beginning an exercise program or participating in exercise testing, you should evaluate your health status to identify any existing medical conditions or risk factors that could be exacerbated by physical activity. The process of evaluation is commonly referred to as a health risk appraisal (HRA). An HRA need not be complex. In fact, the vast majority of medical conditions and risk factors that are predictive of future cardiovascular, orthopaedic and metabolic events can be identified by a well-designed health/medical history questionnaire.

An HRA can be self-administered, provided you have access to an acceptable evaluative instrument and possess an appropriate level of understanding regarding how to interpret the information obtained by the process. In most instances, however, an HRA is conducted by either a medical or a health and fitness professional with training and expertise in the entire evaluative process.

WHY CONDUCT A PRE-ACTIVITY HEALTH APPRAISAL?

For most individuals exercise is a safe endeavor. For a few people, however, exercise can involve some substantial degree of risk. Accordingly, it is advisable that all adults undergo some type of pre-activity HRA before initiating an exercise program and, on a periodic basis thereafter, to identify any subsequent changes in the individual's health status. According to the American College of Sports Medicine (ACSM), a pre-activity HRA is important for a number of reasons, including:

- to identify and exclude individuals with medical contraindications to exercise.

- to assure the safety of exercise testing and exercise programs.
- to determine the appropriate exercise test or exercise program for an individual.
- to identify individuals with clinically significant disease conditions who should be referred to a medically supervised exercise program.
- to identify individuals with either disease symptoms or risk factors for disease who should receive further medical evaluation before initiating an exercise program.
- to identify individuals who have special needs that might preclude them from safely participating in physical activity, such as the elderly, persons with specific orthopaedic conditions, and exercises with pregnancy-related risks.
- to provide information that might serve as the basis of advice given to an individual regarding the relationship between good health and that person's behavior as it relates to physical activity and the risk of developing heart disease, orthopaedic problems, metabolic conditions or other diseases.
- to obtain information to motivate an individual toward meaningful lifestyle changes.

WHAT ARE THE COMPONENTS OF AN HRA?

An HRA should, first and foremost, be valid, cost-effective, easily understood and time-efficient. Self-administered health/medical history questionnaires should be the primary HRA tool used in non-medical (e. g., the majority of health and fitness clubs) facilities. The Physical Activity Readiness Questionnaire (PAR-Q) is an excellent example of a very basic, yet effective, health/medical questionnaire for screening at-risk individuals prior to their participating in exercise (refer to Figure 2-1).

A more comprehensive health/medical history questionnaire (refer to Figure 2-2) usually includes more detailed information concerning an individual's background and current lifestyle, such as data on personal and family history of coronary artery or other diseases and their associated risk factors, current medications, eating habits, smoking history, and current physical activity patterns. The fitness goals and objectives of the individual can also be part of the information collected by the HRA instrument.

In addition to serving as an effective means for gathering medical and lifestyle background information, a well-designed HRA instrument should have the following features:

- it should require responses to questions which are not overly time-consuming (e.g., accordingly, the checklist approach is recommended).
- it should be easily understood.
- it should be simple and straightforward (e.g., individuals should not be required to refer to their medical records).
- it should be updated by the individual on a regular basis (e.g., approximately every six to twelve months).

Figure 2-1. Physical Activity Readiness Questionnaire ("PAR-Q").

PAR-Q & YOU

PAR-Q is designed to help you help yourself. Many health benefits are associated with regular exercise, and the completion of PAR-Q is a sensible first step to take if you are planning to increase the amount of physical activity in your life.

For most people, physical activity should not pose any problem or hazard. PAR-Q has been designed to identify the small number of adults for whom physical activity might be inappropriate or those who should have medical advice concerning the type of activity most suitable for them.

Common sense is your best guide in answering these few questions. Please read them carefully and check the "YES" or "NO" box opposite each question if it applies to you.

YES	NO	
☐	☐	1. Has your doctor ever said you have heart trouble?
☐	☐	2. Do you frequently have pains in your heart and chest?
☐	☐	3. Do you often feel faint or have spells of severe dizziness?
☐	☐	4. Has a doctor ever said your blood pressure was too high?
☐	☐	5. Has your doctor ever told you that you have a bone or joint problem such as arthritis that has been aggravated by exercise, or might be made worse with exercise?
☐	☐	6. Is there a good physical reason not mentioned here why you should not follow an activity program even if you wanted to?
☐	☐	7. Are you over age 65 and not accustomed to vigorous exercise?

 IF YOU ANSWERED:

YES TO ONE OR MORE QUESTIONS:

If you have not recently done so, consult with your physician by telephone or in person BEFORE increasing your physical activity and/or taking a fitness appraisal. Tell your physician what questions you answered YES to on PAR-Q or present your PAR-Q copy.

After medical evaluation, seek advice from your physician as to your suitability for:

• Unrestricted physical activity, starting off easily and progressing gradually.

• Restricted or supervised activity to meet your specific needs, at least on an initial basis. Check in your community for special programs or services.

NO TO ALL QUESTIONS:

If you answered PAR-Q accurately, you have reasonable assurance of your present suitability for:

• A graduated exercise program—a gradual increase in proper exercise promotes good fitness development while minimizing or eliminating discomfort.

• An exercise test—simple tests of fitness (such as the Canadian Home Fitness Test) or more complex types may be undertaken if you so desire.

Remember to postpone physical activity if you have a temporary minor illness, such as a common cold.

Developed by the British Columbia Ministry of Health. Conceptualized and critiqued by the Multidisciplinary Advisory Board on Exercise (MABE). Translation, reproduction and use in its entirety is encouraged.

Figure 2-2. Health/Medical History Questionnaire.

NAME

ADDRESS

PHONE (home) (   )   -   (work) (   )   -

AGE   BIRTH DATE   OCCUPATION

PHYSICIAN'S NAME

PHYSICIAN'S ADDRESS   PHONE

Risk Factor Questionnaire

Yes	No		
❑	❑	1.	Have you ever had, or has your doctor ever diagnosed you as having, heart trouble or coronary disease?
❑	❑	2.	Do you have a family history of heart problems or coronary disease?
❑	❑	3.	Do you have a history of high blood pressure (above 140/90)?
❑	❑	4.	Do you have diabetes?
❑	❑	5.	Do you smoke cigarettes?
❑	❑	6.	Are you overweight?
❑	❑	7.	Is your diet heavy in fatty foods and red meat?
❑	❑	8.	Do you ever have pains in your heart/chest?
❑	❑	9.	Do you ever feel faint or have dizzy spells?
❑	❑	10.	Has your doctor ever said you have high cholesterol?
❑	❑	11.	Are you over 65 and sedentary?
❑	❑	12.	Resting ECG: _____
❑	❑	13.	Total cholesterol/HDL ratio: _____

Health/Fitness History

1. Are you presently involved in a regular exercise program? If yes, please list activity, duration, frequency, and intensity.
2. Do you now or have you ever smoked?   _____ Yes   _____No
   (a) If you previously smoked, how long did you smoke, how often, and when did you quit?
   (b) If you currently smoke, how much?

Figure 2-2. Health/Medical History Questionnaire (cont.)

3. Do you use alcohol? _____Yes _____No
     (a) If yes, how much per day? _____
          How much per week? _____
4. Do you drink coffee or colas with caffeine? _____Yes _____No
     (a) If yes, how much per day?_____
5. Are you now or have you every been on a diet? _____ Yes _____No
     (a) If yes, please explain.
6. Do you consider yourself overweight or underweight? (*please circle*)
7. How many meals do you usually eat per day? _____
8. Do you usually eat breakfast? _____Yes _____No
9. How many eggs do you eat per week? _____
10. How many times per week do you usually eat the following?
     Beef _____ Fish _____ Pork _____ Fowl _____
     Desserts _____ Fried Foods _____ Fast Foods _____
11. Do you regularly use any of the following? (*please circle*)
     Butter   Sugar   Sweeteners   Salt   Whole milk
12. How active do you consider yourself? (*please circle*)
     Sedentary   Lightly active   Moderately active   Highly active
13. How would you describe your nutrition habits? (*please circle*)
     Good   Fair   Poor
14. How would you characterize your life? (*please circle*)
     Highly stressful   Moderately stressful   Low in stress
15. Please describe your knowledge of exercise and fitness. (*please circle*)
     Good   Fair   Poor

16. Please describe your knowledge of nutrition. (*please circle*)
     Good   Fair   Poor

Medical History

Present and past history
1. Check any conditions or diseases you now have or have had in the past.
     ❏   Heart attack, coronary bypass, or other cardiac surgery
     ❏   Diabetes
     ❏   Stroke
     ❏   Peripheral vascular disease
     ❏   Phlebitis or emboli
     ❏   Rheumatic fever
     ❏   High blood pressure
     ❏   Low blood pressure
     ❏   Chest discomfort
     ❏   Extra, skipped, or rapid heart beats or palpitations
     ❏   Heart murmurs
     ❏   Ankle swelling
     ❏   Cold hands or feet
     ❏   Unusual shortness of breath
     ❏   Light-headedness or fainting
     ❏   Epilepsy or seizures
     ❏   Anemia

Figure 2-2. Health/Medical History Questionnaire (cont.)

- ❏ Asthma
- ❏ Emphysema
- ❏ Bronchitis
- ❏ Pneumonia
- ❏ A chronic recurrent cough
- ❏ Increased anxiety or depression
- ❏ Emotional disorders
- ❏ Fatigue or lack of energy
- ❏ Trouble sleeping
- ❏ Migraine or recurrent headaches
- ❏ Swollen, stiff, or painful joints
- ❏ Foot problems
- ❏ Knee problems
- ❏ Back problems
- ❏ Shoulder problems
- ❏ Neck problems
- ❏ Broken bones
- ❏ Ulcers
- ❏ Stomach or intestinal problems
- ❏ Hernia
- ❏ Limited range of motion in joints
- ❏ Arthritis
- ❏ Bursitis

If you checked any of these, please explain.

2.   Please list any prescribed medications you are now taking.

3.   Please list any over-the-counter medications or dietary supplements you are now taking.

4.   Please list any illness, hospitalization, or surgical procedure within the past two years.

5.   Please list any drug allergies.

6.   Please list date of last physical examination and results.

Fitness Goals

Please check specific goals and list dates for achieving them.

- ❏ Improve strength
- ❏ Improve flexibility
- ❏ Improve cardiovascular fitness
- ❏ Improve muscle tone and shape
- ❏ Improve diet/eating habits
- ❏ Lose weight/inches
- ❏ Gain weight/muscle
- ❏ Reduce stress
- ❏ Increase energy
- ❏ Stop smoking/drinking
- ❏ Injury prevention
- ❏ Rehabilitate injury
- ❏ Additional goals (list):

How Should The Information Obtained From An HRA Be Used?

Once the information is obtained and evaluated by someone with an appropriate level of knowledge, you can be classified into the appropriate risk category for possible exercise testing and subsequent participation in physical activity programs. The ACSM proposes the following three major categories for individuals who may desire to undergo an exercise test and/or participate in an exercise program:

- *Apparently healthy*: Those who are asymptomatic and are apparently healthy with no more than one major coronary risk factor (refer to Table 2-1).
- *Individuals at higher risk*: Those who have two or more major coronary risk factors or who have symptoms suggestive of possible cardiopulmonary or metabolic disease (refer to Table 2-2).
- *Individuals with disease*: Those who have documented cardiac, pulmonary or metabolic disease.

Table 2-1. Major Coronary Risk Factors.

1. Cigarette smoking
2. Hypertension (>140/90 mmHg borderline, > 160/95 severe)
3. Hyperlipidemia (total cholesterol > 240 mg/dl or total cholesterol/high density lipoprotein ratio > 4.5)
4. Diabetes mellitus (fasting blood glucose > 140 mg/dl)
5. Heredity family history of coronary disease (in parents or siblings prior to age 55)

Modified from American College of Sports Medicine (1991) and American Heart Association (1988).

In response to a need for general guidelines regarding exercise testing and exercise prescription for individuals in the aforementioned categories, the ACSM developed the following recommendations (refer to Table 2-3):

- *Apparently healthy individuals*: Men below the age of 40 and women below 50 can safely begin moderate-intensity (40%-60% of maximal heart rate reserve) exercise programs without undergoing an exercise test or a medical examination. Individuals in this category can also gradually increase the level of intensity of their workout as long as they exercise on a regular basis.
- *Individuals at high risk*: Individuals classified as being at higher risk who are asymptomatic can engage in moderate-intensity exercise without undergoing an exercise test or a medical examination if the exercise is undertaken gradually and is supervised by qualified exercise professionals.

• *Individuals with disease*: Individuals who have a disease which has been documented (cardiac, pulmonary or metabolic) should be referred to their physician for appropriate medical clearance before being allowed to participate in any physical activity program. Their physician should also be requested to identify any exercise limitations or restrictions for these individuals.

Table 2-2. Major Symptoms or Signs Suggestive of Cardiopulmonary or Metabolic Disease*.

---

1. Pain or discomfort in the chest or surrounding areas that appears to be ischemic in nature
2. Unaccustomed shortness of breath or shortness of breath with mild exertion
3. Dizziness or fainting spells
4. Difficult or labored breathing—especially sudden episodes during sleep
5. Ankle swelling
6. Irregular heart beats or accelerated heart rate
7. Severe intermittent leg pain
8. Known heart murmur

---

* These symptoms must be interpreted in the clinical context in which they appear, since they are not all specific for cardiopulmonary or metabolic disease.

Modified from American College of Sports Medicine (1991).

SAFETY ABOVE ALL ELSE

For years, many professionals in the medical community have ascribed to three basic rules for rehabilitating their patients, which also have direct application for individuals who want to engage in a sound exercise program:

Rule #1. Create an environment for optimal healing.
Rule #2. Above all else, DO NO HARM.
Rule #3. Be as aggressive as you can, without breaking Rule #2.

Obviously, all of the positive benefits of exercise will be inconsequential to you if your safety is compromised by the activity. In order to minimize the possibility that such an event might occur, an appropriate HRA should be administered prior to engaging in any type of exercise test or physical activity program for the first time.

An HRA is a tool whose primary purpose is to help protect you from experiencing any serious untoward events during your participation in exercise. The basic objective of pre-activity screening is not diagnostic, but rather to determine risk, whether it be cardiovascular, orthopaedic, metabolic, etc. An HRA, if properly used, should be able to:

- determine if you have a medical condition or risk factor that could be exacerbated by exercise.
- be used to develop appropriate exercise tests and prescriptions.
- be used to educate and motivate you to initiate and sustain necessary lifestyle behavioral changes.

Table 2-3. Guidelines for Exercise Testing and Participation.

	Apparently Healthy		Higher Risk*		
	Younger ≤ 40 yrs. (men ≤ 50 yrs. (women)	Older	No Symptoms	Symptoms	With Disease
Medical exam and diagnostic exercise test recommended prior to:					
Moderate exercise ≠	No§	No	No	Yes	Yes
Vigorous exercise #	No	Yes**	Yes	Yes	Yes
Physician supervision recommended during exercise test:					
Sub-maximal testing	No	No	No	Yes	Yes
Maximal testing	No	Yes	Yes	Yes	Yes

*   Persons with two or more risk factors (refer to Table 2-1) or symptoms (refer to Table 2-2).

=   Persons with known cardiac, pulmonary, or metabolic disease.

≠   Moderate exercise (exercise intensity 40 to 60% $\dot{V}O_2$ max)—Exercise intensity well within the individual's current capacity and can be comfortably sustained for a prolonged period of time, i.e., 60 minutes, slow progression, and generally non-competitive.

\#   Vigorous exercise (exercise intensity > 60% $\dot{V}O_2$ max)—Exercise intense enough to represent a substantial challenge and which would ordinarily result in fatigue within 20 minutes.

§   The "no" responses in this table mean that an item is "not necessary." The "no" response does **not** mean that the item should not be done.

**   A "yes" response means that an item is recommended.

From American College of Sports Medicine : Guidelines for Exercise Testing and Prescription, 4th ed. Philadelphia, Lea & Febiger, 1991. Reprinted with permission.

Given the many desirable consequences of sound exercise, it is sometimes too easy and too convenient to jump right into an exercise program without spending a few moments to ensure that your safety will not be compromised by the endeavor. Accordingly, an HRA should be viewed as a user-friendly form of "safety insurance." ❏

BIBLIOGRAPHY •

1. American College of Sports Medicine. *ACSM's Health/Fitness Facility Standards and Guidelines*. Champaign, IL: Human Kinetics Publishers, 1992.
2. American College of Sports Medicine. *Guidelines for Exercise Testing and Prescription*, 4th Ed. Philadelphia, PA: Lea & Febiger, 1991.
3. American Heart Association. *1988 Heart Facts*. Dallas, TX: American Heart Association, 1988.
4. Chisholm, D.M., Collis, M.L., Kulak, L.L., et al. "Physical activity readiness." *Br Col Med J* 17:375-378, 1975.
5. Fardy, P.S., Yanowitz, F.G., Wilson, P.K. *Cardiac Rehabilitation, Adult Fitness, and Exercise Testing*, 2nd Ed. Philadelphia, PA: Lea & Febiger, 1988.
6. Howley, E.T., Franks, B.D. *Health Fitness Instructor's Handbook*, 2nd Ed. Champaign, IL: Human Kinetics Publishers, 1992.
7. Koeberle, B.E. *Legal Aspects of Sports Medicine*. Canton, OH: Professional Reports Corporation, 1990.
8. Nieman, D.C. *Fitness and Sports Medicine: An Introduction*. Palo Alto, CA: Bull Publishing Company, 1990.
9. Shephard, R.J. "PAR-Q, Canadian home fitness test and exercise screening alternatives." *Sports Med* 5:185-195, 1988.

CHAPTER 3

· ·

ASSESSING AND ADDRESSING CORONARY RISK FACTORS

by

Wayne L. Westcott, Ph.D.
James L. Hodgson, Ph.D.
and
W. Channing Nicholas, M.D.

· · ·

*H*eart disease is the leading cause of death in the United States. In 1990, according to the American Heart Association, almost 800,000 Americans died from heart disease. This catastrophic total can be better understood when it is compared to the total number of Americans who died in World War I (116,516), World War II (405,399), Korea (54,246), Vietnam (58,000) and the Persian Gulf (290) collectively—634,451 deaths. In the decade of the 1980s, more than 7,000,000 Americans died from some form of cardiovascular disease.

Fortunately, EXERCISE—particularly aerobic exercise—can help prevent you from becoming a victim of heart and vascular disease. Heart disease is not the inevitable consequence of aging. Research has shown that lifestyle is a major contributing factor to heart disease. Too much saturated fat. Too much sodium. Too much alcohol. Too much smoking. Too much body weight. Not enough exercise.

By ignoring the muscle that may matter most in the body—the heart—and using the major chewing muscle (masseter) that needs the least attention, we expose ourselves to the deadly risks of cardiovascular disease. The more we abuse our bodies and the more we ignore the need to have a healthy heart, the greater the likelihood we'll suffer from heart and vascular disease.

Probably, the most serious form of vascular disease is coronary artery disease (CAD). Nearly one-third of all of the non-accidental deaths that occur in the United States each year result from CAD. Essentially, CAD involves the obstruction of the blood supply to the heart through the three major coronary arteries. The narrowing, hardening, and blocking of these arteries through the buildup of lipids in the inner layers of these arteries lead to CAD. Eventually, the coronary artery is occluded to a point where part of the heart muscle does not get enough blood (oxygen and nutrients) and the individual suffers a heart attack (i.e., part of the heart muscle dies). The serious nature of heart attacks is reflected in the fact that more than one out of three individuals die from their <u>first</u> heart attack and that more than 300,000 Americans die annually from a heart attack <u>before</u> reaching the hospital.

An obvious question arises: What can be done to reduce an individual's risk for heart disease? A number of extensive clinical studies have identified the major risk factors for heart disease. Although not an inclusive listing, eight factors that account for a large portion of the heart disease in the United States are listed in Table 3-1. An individual's chance of getting heart disease and suffering a heart attack increases with the number of risk factors present.

Table 3-1. Significant Risk Factors for Heart Disease.

- Family history of coronary heart disease (before age 55)
- Cigarette smoking (an individual smokes more than ten cigarettes per day)
- Hypercholesterolemia (an individual's total blood cholesterol level is too high—equal to or greater than 240 mg/dl; and/or the level of the "bad" low density lipoprotein cholesterol is too high (≥ 130 mg/dl) or the "good" high density lipoprotein cholesterol level in your blood is too low (below 35 mg/dl)
- Hypertension (an individual's systolic blood pressure is ≥ 160 mm Hg and/or diastolic blood pressure is ≥ 90 mm Hg)
- Diabetes mellitus (an individual's fasting blood glucose—sugar—levels are ≥ 140 mg/dl)
- Severe obesity (a body fat level ≥ 25% for men or ≥ 30% for women)
- Stressful lifestyle
- Sedentary lifestyle

FAMILY HISTORY OF CORONARY HEART DISEASE OR DIABETES

A positive family history of coronary heart disease is undoubtedly one of the most serious risk factors for heart disease. Regrettably, if you a strong family history of cardiovascular disease, nothing can change what you have inherited. The good news is that knowledge is power, and you can concentrate on those risk factors which can be modified. It is, therefore, extremely important for persons with an unfavorable medical family history (parents, brothers or sisters) to reduce all of the other known coronary risk factors as much as possible. It is equally essential that they have regular and comprehensive medical checkups by a physician to identify any potential problems at the earliest and most treatable stages.

CIGARETTE SMOKING

In addition to causing several types of cancer and a variety of other fatal diseases, cigarette smoking is a potent coronary risk factor. Without detailing the numerous medical consequences of cigarette smoking, almost everyone agrees that smoking presents a very serious health hazard. However, good news exists for smokers. Smokers who stop smoking eventually lower their coronary risk to almost the same level as persons who have never smoked.

Although the number of carefully controlled scientific research studies in this area are somewhat lacking, considerable empirical evidence exists to support the contention that most smokers do not engage in regular exercise, and that most regular exercisers do *NOT* smoke. Exceptions exist to this observation, but a good case could be made that regular exercise and smoking may be mutually exclusive behaviors. Without question, all individuals who currently smoke should be strongly encouraged to develop and engage in a sound exercise program. It may very well provide the individual a higher level of satisfaction than smoking, and serve as a powerful incentive to give up an unhealthy addiction.

ELEVATED BLOOD CHOLESTEROL

The amount of cholesterol circulating in the blood has a direct relationship to the accumulation of fatty deposits inside the arteries. Consequently, the higher the cholesterol level, the higher the risk of coronary artery disease.

The first step in dealing with blood cholesterol is having it checked on a routine basis. If the blood cholesterol level of a person is above 240 mg/dl, then that individual is placed in the high risk category according to the United States Public Health Service guidelines. If it is between 200 mg/dl and 240 mg/dl, then that person is categorized as having a moderate risk of CAD; and if it is below 200 mg/dl, then that person is placed in the low risk category for CAD.

Outside of genetic factors, the total blood cholesterol reading is most influenced by a person's nutritional habits. As a general rule, eating less dietary fat (especially saturated fat) will result in lower blood cholesterol levels. As a result, the reduced fat intake diet is probably the most popularly prescribed intervention strategy. However, total cholesterol is composed of two major components known as low-density lipoproteins (LDL cholesterol) and high-density lipoproteins (HDL cholesterol). LDL cholesterol is often referred to as "bad" cholesterol because it accumulates inside the arteries. HDL cholesterol is typically called "good" cholesterol because it helps to move fats quickly out of the bloodstream.

While exercise does not appear to lower an individual's level of total cholesterol (except when it is accompanied by significant weight loss), it has been shown to significantly increase the level of HDL (good) cholesterol. Because higher levels of HDL cholesterol are associated with a lower risk of coronary artery disease, regular exercise may be an effective means for reducing this risk factor.

ELEVATED BLOOD PRESSURE

Elevated blood pressure has long been recognized as a major risk factor for coronary artery disease. Basically, blood pressure is the force exerted by the circulating blood against the artery walls. Blood pressure readings are usually expressed in terms of two numeric values. The higher number represents the arterial pressure during the contraction phase of the heart and is called systolic pressure. The lower number represents the arterial pressure during the relaxation phase of the heart and is called diastolic pressure. All individuals should have their blood pressure checked on a regular basis. A normal resting blood pressure is in the neighborhood of 120/80 mm Hg. Readings above 140 mm Hg systolic or 90 mm Hg diastolic are considered on the high side.

High blood pressure readings are a clear signal that remedial measures must be undertaken. Due to the potential health problems associated with excessive blood pressure, it is essential to take whatever steps may be necessary to bring it into normal range. Intervention strategies usually include taking physician prescribed medications, reducing sodium (salt) consumption, losing body fat, avoiding stressful situations, and performing regular exercise.

A number of studies have demonstrated that regular exercise may be effective for normalizing elevated blood pressures. Although the precise process responsible for this adaptation is not well understood by exercise scientists and physicians, regular exercise has been found to have a positive antihypertensive effect (i.e., lowers blood pressure). Recent studies have shown that regular moderate exercise reduces fatalities due to coronary heart disease in people with elevated blood pressure. Individuals with high blood pressure should be strongly advised prior to initiating an exercise program to first consult their physician.

DIABETES MELLITUS

Approximately one out of every ten American adults is diabetic or displays some form of glucose intolerance. According to the American College of Sports Medicine, diabetes is a major coronary risk factor and contributes to a great many other health problems. Two principal types of diabetes exist: Type I (insulin dependent or juvenile-onset) and Type II (non-insulin dependent or adult-onset). The most prominent characteristic of either form of diabetes is an elevated blood sugar level (hyperglycemia). Hyperglycemia results from insufficient insulin production by the pancreas in Type I diabetes, and from peripheral tissue insensitivity (unresponsiveness) to insulin in Type II diabetes. Regular physical activity has long been shown to be beneficial for diabetics—particularly Type II. Considerable controversy exists, however, regarding how exercise can best be incorporated into the total treatment program for diabetics (for more detailed information regarding exercise programming for diabetics, refer to items 6 and 13 in the bibliography for this chapter).

Obesity

Individuals who carry 20 percent more fat weight than is desirable have a significantly higher risk of coronary artery disease. It is important to realize that an individual's body weight is not as important as that person's relative body composition. Body composition refers to the two major components of body weight—fat weight and lean weight (muscle, bone, organ). Generally speaking, males should be about 15 percent fat and females should be approximately 20 percent fat. Persons who are considerably above these levels (men above 25% and women above 30% are considered to be obese) should take three simple steps to improve their body composition and reduce their coronary risk.

The first step is to reduce the amount of fat foods in their daily diet. Fats present a two-dimensional problem. They tend to elevate blood cholesterol levels, and they contain over twice as many calories per gram as carbohydrates and proteins. Consequently, a decrease in fat intake offers a double benefit to the individual—lower cholesterol levels and reduced caloric intake.

The second step is to perform regular aerobic endurance exercise to burn extra calories and to improve cardiovascular fitness. Vigorous aerobic activities, such as stair climbing, running, cycling and swimming, may burn up to 20 calories per minute while they are being performed. The overweight individual should, however, start with exercise intensities that are much lower (five to eight calories per minute) and over a period of several weeks build up to higher intensities.

The third step is to engage in sensible strength exercise to add muscle tissue and to improve muscular fitness. Because muscle is a very metabolically active tissue, more muscle requires more energy throughout the day for the ongoing repair and rebuilding processes. In fact, it is estimated that every pound of muscle added to the human frame elicits the expenditure of an additional 50 calories per day for tissue maintenance.

Body composition can be reasonably approximated by carefully looking in a full length mirror, but more accurate assessment exists. The more commonly used methods are skinfold calipers, circumference measurements, electrical impedance devices, ultrasound analyzers and underwater weighing. The exact technique used depends on the equipment available and the degree of accuracy desired—some methods are more accurate than others.

Stressful Lifestyle

The extent of the research effort into the possible relationship between CAD and a stressful lifestyle is somewhat limited. Most authorities on the subject consider a stressful lifestyle to be a significant risk factor for coronary artery disease. People with time-conscious, hard-driving, pressure-packed personalities have been shown to be particularly susceptible to heart disease.

Since it may not always be possible to change either the environment or the personality traits of an individual, regular exercise is recommended as a way to dissipate the stress that one can encounter on a daily basis. Research has found that exercise is an excellent means for reducing the overall level of daily stress that individuals face, as well as for "recharging" individuals to enable them to deal with the demands of living and working in our fast-paced society.

SEDENTARY LIFESTYLE

Some experts contend that a sedentary lifestyle is possibly the most problematic coronary risk factor. Sedentary lifestyle is essentially a daily routine that rarely includes any vigorous physical activity. According to the United States Public Health Service, approximately 60 percent of all Americans are sedentary. Even more discouraging, sedentary behavior carries almost the same risk of coronary artery disease as cigarette smoking, high blood pressure, or obesity.

Because sedentary lifestyle is so common and so debilitating, individuals should be strongly urged not to ignore this particular risk factor. In fact, engaging in an active lifestyle has been shown to be an effective means for reducing almost every other coronary risk factor. The potential relationship between regular exercise and many of the primary coronary risk factors can better be understood by reviewing the following list of the beneficial consequences of an active lifestyle:

- Most smokers do not perform regular exercise, and most regular exercisers do not smoke.
- Regular exercise typically increases HDL (good) cholesterol which reduces the risk of fat accumulation inside the arteries. In fact, exercise is one of the few voluntary activities that is effective in raising an individual's level of HDL.
- Regular exercise tends to reduce blood pressure in persons who have elevated blood pressure levels and minimize the deleterious affects of high blood pressure.
- Regular exercise is perhaps the best long term approach for achieving and maintaining desirable body weight. Research has found that obese people have more of the typical risk factors for heart disease (high blood pressure, diabetes and elevated serum cholesterol levels), and they die from it at a substantially higher rate.
- Regular exercise may provide a positive and productive outlet for the stresses often associated with daily living. Exercise dissipates those hormones and other chemicals which build up during periods of high stress. Exercise also generates a period of substantial emotional and physical relaxation that sets in approximately an hour and a half after an intense workout.
- Regular exercise eliminates a sedentary lifestyle, which in itself reduces an individual's level of coronary risk. Experts have found that non-exercisers have twice the risk of developing heart disease than individuals who exercise regularly.

Heart Smart

The key to reducing coronary risk factors is awareness. First, the initial critical step requires that individuals learn where they stand with regard to the various risk factors for heart disease. Then, they need to take the necessary steps to improve their personal health and fitness, as discussed in the previous sections of this chapter. Coronary risk factor assessments should be viewed as mandates for a positive lifestyle change, rather than as condemnation reports. Fortunately, in most instances, individuals can significantly improve their coronary risk profiles. Individuals should keep in mind one fundamental fact: *EVERYONE CAN DO SOMETHING TO LOWER THEIR RISK OF DEVELOPING CARDIO-VASCULAR DISEASE.* Exercise regularly. While it's not 100 percent foolproof, it does offer a great opportunity for a healthy, long life. Surely, everyone deserves no less. ❏

BIBLIOGRAPHY •

1. American College of Sports Medicine. *Guidelines for Exercise Testing and Prescription,* 4th Ed. Philadelphia, PA: Lea & Febiger, 1991.
2. American Heart Association. *1989 Heart Facts.* Dallas, TX: Author, 1989.
3. Blair, S.N., Kohl, H.W., Paffenbarger, R.S., et al. "Physical fitness and all-cause mortality: A prospective study of healthy men and women." *JAMA* 262:2395-2401, 1989.
4. Bouchard, C., Shephard, R.J., Stephens, T., et al. (Eds). *Exercise, Fitness, and Health.* Champaign, IL: Human Kinetics Publishers, 1990.
5. Ekelund, L.G., Haskell, W.L., Johnson, J.L., et al. "Physical fitness as a predictor of cardiovascular mortality in asymptomatic North American men: The Lipid Research Clinics Mortality Follow-up Study." *N Engl J Med* 319:1379-1384, 1988.
6. Franklin, B.A., Gordon, S., Timmis, G.C. (Eds). *Exercise in Modern Medicine.* Baltimore, MD: Williams & Wilkins, 1989.
7. Hubert, H.D., Feinleib, M., McNamara, P.M., et al. "Obesity as an independent risk factor for cardiovascular disease: A 26-year follow-up of participants in the Framingham heart study." *Circulation* 67:968-977, 1983.
8. Joint National Committee. "The 1988 report of the Joint National Committee on detection, evaluation, and treatment of high blood pressure." *Arch Intern Med* 148(5):1023-1038, 1988.
9. National Cholesterol Education Program. "Report of the National Cholesterol Education Program expert panel on detection, evaluation, and treatment of high blood cholesterol in adults." *Arch Intern Med* 148(1):36-69, 1988.
10. National Institute of Health Consensus Development Panel. "Health implications of obesity: National Institute of Health consensus development conference statement." *Ann Intern Med* 103:1073-1077, 1985.
11. Paffenbarger, R.S., Hyde, R.T., Wing, A., et al. "Physical activity, all-cause mortality, and longevity of college alumni." *N Engl J Med* 314:605-613, 1986.
12. Skinner, J.S. (Ed). Exercise Testing and Exercise Prescription for Special Cases. Philadelphia, PA: Lea & Febiger, 1987.
13. The Pooling Project Research Group. "Relationship of blood pressure, serum cholesterol, smoking habit, relative weight and ECG abnormalities to incidence of major coronary events: Final report of the pooling project. *J Chronic Dis* 31(4):201-306, 1978.

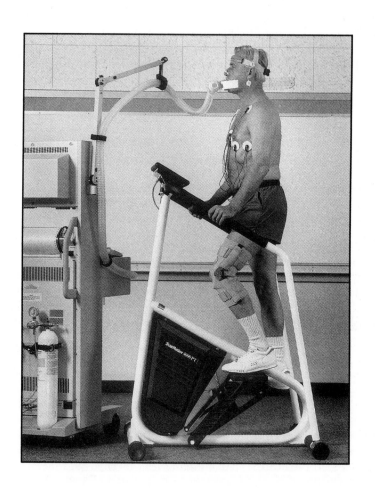

CHAPTER 4

UNDERSTANDING THE PHYSIOLOGICAL BASIS OF CARDIORESPIRATORY FITNESS*

by

James S. Skinner, Ph.D.

• • •

Muscles involved in exercise produce a significant amount of energy by combining foodstuffs with oxygen. As the oxygen needs of your exercising muscles increase, your lungs supply more oxygen to the blood, perfusing them. Your heart, in turn, pumps more oxygenated blood to your working muscles. If a steady supply of oxygen is not produced to meet the energy demands of the activity, then an energy imbalance develops, blood lactate (LA) levels rise, blood pH decreases, and fatigue occurs. Your ability to engage in sustained high levels of physical activity without significant fatigue is determined by the your body's ability to deliver oxygenated blood to your muscles, and the ability of your muscles to extract the oxygen from the blood and utilize it for the production of energy in the form of adenosine triphosphate (ATP). If you're really interested in having a fundamental knowledge of how your body works during different types of exercise, you need to understand both the basic concepts of energy production and the physiological adjustments made by your body to meet the increased energy requirements of exercising skeletal muscles.

BASIC CONCEPTS OF ENERGY AND ITS SOURCES

The energy that is required for the normal functioning (muscle contraction, conduction of nervous impulses, hormone synthesis, etc.) of every living cell in your body is produced by chemical reactions. These chemical reactions are either

---

*Note: Some of the material contained in this chapter is adapted from *Body Energy* by James S. Skinner, 1981 (Anderson World Inc., Mountain View, CA).

aerobic (occurring in the presence of oxygen) or anaerobic (without oxygen). You must continually produce energy or the various tissues and organs in your body will cease to function. It would be akin to pulling out the plug of an electric appliance.

To clarify the relationship between food consumption and energy production, you should think of your body as a factory. It must process different raw materials to make its final product—energy. This energy is used by every cell of your body. The three basic raw materials your body uses to produce energy are oxygen, carbohydrates (sugar and starches) and fat. These materials essentially are available in an unlimited supply. Since we live in a veritable sea of oxygen, an adequate supply is generally not a problem. When you eat food, you replenish the other raw materials your body needs to produce energy.

Under normal circumstances, your body does not directly use protein for energy production. Proteins provide much of the structural basis for cells and are a major component of enzymes (substances responsible for controlling various chemical reactions at the cellular level). If you consume more protein than your body needs, the excess will be converted into fat or carbohydrate.

Since the amount of energy required at rest is so small, your body doesn't consume much oxygen. Accordingly, your resting energy needs are easily met by your aerobic system. During the initial stages of exercise, however, the situation changes. When the work demands placed on your body increase, your body needs extra energy immediately. Unfortunately, the rate of aerobic energy production is sluggish (i.e., oxygen must be breathed in, transferred from your lungs to the blood, carried to your heart and then pumped to your muscles where it actually is needed). Thus, a delay exists in the delivery of oxygen from the outside. If a sudden demand for more energy arises, an emergency back-up system must exist that will permit your body to function until the aerobic "assembly line" speeds up its production. The anaerobic energy system serves this function.

A given amount of work requires a given amount of energy. The following descriptive time table illustrates how energy is produced during the initial stages of exercise and during mild exercise.

- When exercise first starts, only a limited supply of energy is present in the muscle for immediate use—during this phase, oxygen is not required.
- Either glycogen stored in the muscle or glucose transported by the blood from the liver can be used without oxygen to provide a limited supply of energy. Lactic acid is the by-product of this anaerobic reaction.
- Most of the lactic acid formed during an anaerobic reaction is released into the blood and transported to the liver, where it is converted back to glycogen and stored.
- As additional oxygen becomes available, the aerobic system is used more and more. After a few minutes, the aerobic system is able to supply all the energy needed for mild exercise.

- At this time, liver glycogen is converted to glucose and released into the blood to provide fuel for both systems (aerobic and anaerobic).
- Finally, adipocytes (fat cells) release more and more fat, the preferred fuel for the aerobic system.

If the exercise bout is intense, other events take place to ensure that adequate amounts of energy are provided for your working skeletal muscles. The production of energy during exercise of high intensity occurs as follows:

- The speed of the aerobic reactions increases to provide more energy—more carbon dioxide is also produced.
- The faster anaerobic system supplies increasing amounts of energy as the exercise becomes more intense. The intensity of the muscle contractions causes a compression of the small arteries and no oxygen, glucose or fat can enter the muscle cell. Thus, the majority of the carbohydrate needed comes from that which is already stored within the muscle itself.
- Eventually, more lactic acid is formed and increased amounts of lactic acid are released into the bloodstream. As lactic acid levels within the muscle increase, the efficiency of the aerobic chemical reactions are inhibited. When this occurs, inadequate amounts of energy can be produced aerobically. Accordingly, you have to either slow down (reduce the amount of energy needed) or rely more heavily on your anaerobic system.
- Only a small percentage of lactic acid is transformed back into glycogen in the liver; the majority remains in the blood and the muscles. Your body can accumulate and tolerate a limited amount of lactic acid. In all likelihood, it is the presence of lactic acid that causes you to breathe excessively, experience feelings of fatigue and heaviness in your muscles and forces you eventually to stop exercising.

To better understand the relative importance of the anaerobic and aerobic systems for energy production, refer to Figure 4-1. This figure provides an approximate idea of the maximal amount of energy a well-trained individual can produce over time, and how that energy is produced. For comparison purposes, the energy required at rest is given a value of one.

Although the stored energy can be used very rapidly, and individuals can perform a lot of work, these stockpiles are essentially exhausted after ten to twenty seconds. This partially explains why individuals cannot run 400 meters as fast as they can 100 meters, or why weight lifters can lift more in one lift than they can in three lifts without a pause.

The production of energy anaerobically is relatively high, peaking at around 40 to 50 seconds. It doesn't last long because you are limited by your body's tolerance of lactic acid. After 10 minutes, the amount of energy produced by this mechanism is very small.

After five to six minutes of continuous exercise, the majority of energy your body requires has to be produced aerobically. The longer the duration of exercise, the greater the importance of the aerobic system. Anything over ten minutes has to be performed aerobically, except for occasional, brief increases in work output.

Table 4-1. Relative importance of various energy-producing systems over time.

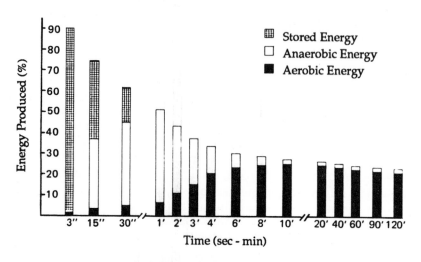

Used with permission from Body Energy by James S. Skinner, 1981 (Anderson World Inc., Mountain View, CA).

MAXIMAL OXYGEN UPTAKE

If you increase the intensity of exercise, a number of things happen in your body. A rise occurs in heart rate, respiration, and oxygen intake, as well as in the activity levels of other parts of your oxygen delivery and utilization (aerobic) systems. A point occurs, however, beyond which oxygen intake cannot increase, even though more work is being performed. At this point, you have reached a level that is commonly referred to as maximal oxygen uptake ($\dot{V}O_2$ max). This is considered to be the best single indicator of cardiorespiratory fitness, since it involves the optimal ability of three major systems (pulmonary, cardiovascular, and muscular) of your body to take in, transport and utilize oxygen. Thus, the higher your level of maximal oxygen uptake, the greater your level of physical working capacity.

THE RELATIONSHIP BETWEEN THE PRODUCTION OF ENERGY AND THE INTENSITY OF EXERCISE

If the amount of work being performed is progressively increased, at some work output along the continuum as you approach your level of maximum capacity, your ability to produce energy aerobically will not be able to completely match your energy demands. For most sedentary people, this occurs at a work output requiring approximately half of their $\dot{V}O_2$ max. In other words, below 50% $\dot{V}O_2$ max, the "slower" aerobic system can provide all the energy that you need. Of course, your body does not switch over to the anaerobic system all at once, but gradually shifts gears to produce energy at a faster rate. A level between 50% and 70% $\dot{V}O_2$ max represents a transition phase for most people. Above 70% $\dot{V}O_2$ max, your aerobic system does not produce energy fast enough causing you to rely more and more on your anaerobic system.

Figure 4-2 is a schematic diagram of the level of lactic acid in the blood relative to the intensity of exercise. The level of lactic acid is a rough indicator of the degree to which you are using the anaerobic mechanism. As the diagram illustrates, lactic acid will begin to rise slowly around 50% $\dot{V}O_2$ max. Up to 70% of maximum, because the increase is not too great, your body can compensate with little trouble. Beyond 70% $\dot{V}O_2$ max, however, as the buildup of lactic acid becomes more dramatic, you will start to get "winded." This explains why you can run at a certain pace (50% to 60% $\dot{V}O_2$ max) with no problem, but become exhausted quickly after trying to run faster (80% to 90% $\dot{V}O_2$ max).

Table 4-2. Lactic acid in the blood related to exercise intensity.

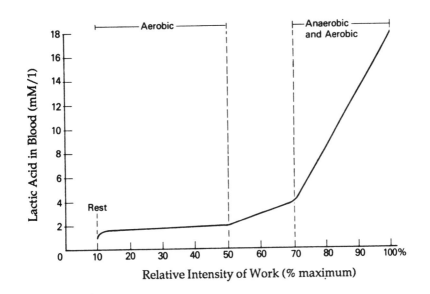

Used with permission from Body Energy by James S. Skinner, 1981 (Anderson World Inc., Mountain View, CA).

Depending on the intensity and duration levels of the activity, most sporting activities require both aerobic and anaerobic production of energy. For example, soccer players perform aerobic exercise when running for twenty to thirty minutes nonstop. Of course, if the activity did not depend on the aerobic system for energy, they would not be able to run for nearly so long. Occasionally, soccer players must sprint after the ball. During those high-intensity intervals, which exceed 70% of their $\dot{V}O_2$ max, they are forced to draw upon their emergency, anaerobic sources. Anaerobic chemical reactions are primarily used in high-intensity exercise of relatively brief duration (e.g., sprinting short distances or heavy weight lifting), while aerobic chemical reactions are primarily involved in low-intensity, long-duration exercise activities such as walking, cycling, stair climbing, etc.

PHYSIOLOGICAL ADJUSTMENTS TO EXERCISE

The aerobic metabolism of fats and carbohydrates is the preferred and more efficient mode of energy production. It, however, can be limited by your body's ability to transport and deliver oxygen to, and the utilization of oxygen by, your working muscles. Several physiological adjustments are made during exercise. The primary objective of these adjustments is to provide an exercising muscle with oxygenated blood that can be used for the production of energy. Your endurance capabilities will be greatly influenced by the magnitude and direction of these changes.

CARDIAC OUTPUT

The amount of blood pumped per minute by your heart is termed your cardiac output ($\dot{Q}$). This measure is indicative of the rate of oxygen delivery to your peripheral tissues (e.g., exercising skeletal muscles). Cardiac output, which is the product of heart rate (HR) and stroke volume (SV), increases linearly as a function of work rate. At rest, $\dot{V}O_2$ is roughly five liters per minute (an average value for males), but can rise to 20-25 liters per minute during exercise in young, healthy adults. This exercise-induced increase of $\dot{Q}$ is due to alterations in both HR and SV.

HEART RATE

Heart rate, one of the two primary determinants of $\dot{Q}$, also rises linearly with work rate. The gradual withdrawal of vagal (parasympathetic nervous system) influences and the progressive increases in sympathetic nerve activity which occur during exercise are largely responsible for the observed increases in HR. At or near $\dot{V}O_2$ max, HR begins to level off and is referred to as maximal heart rate. The equation "220 minus your age" (expressed in whole years) provides a rough estimate of your maximal heart rate (with a standard deviation of 10 to 12 beats per minute). As the equation implies, your maximal heart rate declines with age.

STROKE VOLUME

Stroke volume is the other primary determinant of Q and represents the amount of blood ejected from the heart during each beat. Unlike HR, SV does not increase linearly with work rate. SV increases progressively until a work rate equivalent to approximately 50-75% $\dot{V}O_2$ max is reached. Thereafter, continued increases in work rate cause little or no increase in SV. Exercise-induced increases in SV are believed to be the result of factors that are both intrinsic and extrinsic to the heart. According to the Frank-Starling law, a greater stretch is placed on the muscle fibers of the heart (due to a greater venous return of blood to the heart), resulting in a more forceful contraction of those fibers and consequently a greater SV. Extrinsic factors such as increased nervous (sympathetic) or endocrine (release of adrenal hormones epinephrine and norepinephrine) stimulation to the myocardium can also contribute to the increased SV that occurs during exercise.

BLOOD PRESSURE

Systolic blood pressure (SBP) represents the force developed by your heart during ventricular contraction. SBP increases linearly with work rate. In healthy adults, SBP tends not to exceed 220 mm Hg at maximal exercise levels (according to the American College of Sports Medicine, 250 mm Hg should be considered an end point for a maximal exercise test). Diastolic blood pressure (DBP) is indicative of the pressure in the arterial system during ventricular relaxation and reflects peripheral resistance to blood flow. It changes little from rest to maximal levels of exercise. Therefore, the pulse pressure (the algebraic difference between SBP and DBP) increases in direct proportion to the intensity of exercise. The pulse pressure is important since it reflects the driving force for blood flow in the arteries.

TOTAL PERIPHERAL RESISTANCE

The sum of all the forces that oppose blood flow in the systemic circulation is called the total peripheral resistance (TPR). Numerous factors can affect TPR, including blood viscosity, vessel length, hydrostatic pressure, and vessel diameter. Vessel diameter is by far the most important of these factors, since TPR is inversely proportional to the fourth power of the radius of the vessel. If one vessel has one-half the radius of another and if all other factors are equal, the larger vessel would have 16 times (2^4) less resistance than the smaller vessel. As a result, 16 times more blood would flow through the larger vessel at the same pressure. This has important implications for exercise, since certain organs require more blood flow than others during physical activity. During exercise, resistance in the vessels supplying the muscle and skin is decreased (this implies that blood flow to these parts of the body is enhanced), while resistance in vessels supplying visceral organs (e.g., the liver, GI tract, kidneys) is increased (blood flow is reduced). These changes are almost entirely due to intrinsic factors (the increased metabolic demand of the muscle and the requirement of skin blood flow to facilitate heat dissipation). The TPR tends to decrease during progressive dynamic exercise, because vasodilation occurring in the muscle and skin seem to override the vasoconstriction which is occurring in the visceral organs.

ARTERIOVENOUS OXYGEN DIFFERENCE

The arteriovenous oxygen difference, as its name implies, is the difference between the oxygen contents of the arterial blood and mixed venous blood. It is a reflection of the amount of oxygen extracted from your blood by your muscles. The oxygen content of venous blood can be reduced to one-half to one-third the resting levels by exercising muscles, indicative that your muscles are extracting a much higher proportion of the oxygen delivered to them in the arterial blood (approximately 85% of the oxygen in arterial blood can be removed during maximal exercise).

ENERGY IS THE KEY

The physiological adjustments of the cardiovascular and muscular systems are essential to determining your ability to sustain low resistance, dynamic physical activity (i.e., cardiorespiratory fitness level). These adjustments, as discussed in this chapter, support the increased energy requirements associated with exercise. The Fick equation ($\dot{V}O_2 = \dot{Q} \times a\text{-}vO_2$ difference) illustrates how your cardiovascular and muscular systems adjust to supply oxygen to exercising muscles. As the oxygen requirements of your muscles increase, your cardiovascular system responds by elevating HR and SV. Concurrently, your muscular system responds by extracting more oxygen from the blood. For the majority of individuals, oxygen uptake primarily is dependent upon the delivery of oxygen to, and utilization of oxygen by, the exercising muscles. ❑

BIBLIOGRAPHY •

1. Astrand, P.O., Rodahl, K. *Textbook of Work Physiology*, 3rd Ed. New York, NY: McGraw-Hill, 1986.
2. Brooks, G.A., Fahey, T.D. *Exercise Physiology: Human Bioenergetics and Its Applications*. New York, NY: John Wiley & Sons, 1984.
3. Burke, E., Cerny, F., Costill D., et al. "Characteristics of skeletal muscle in competitive cyclists." *Med Sci Sports* 9:109-112, 1977.
4. Chapman, C.B., Mitchell, J.H. "The physiology of exercise." *Sci Am* 212(5):88-96, 1965.
5. Costill, D., Daniels, J., Evans, W., et al. "Skeletal muscle enzymes and fiber composition in male and female track athletes." *J Appl Physiol* 40:149-154, 1976.
6. Fox, E.L., Bowers, R.D., Foss, M.L. *The Physiological Basis of Physical Education and Athletics*, 4th Ed. Philadelphia, PA: W. B. Saunders Company, 1988.
7. Gollnick, P., Armstrong, R., Saubert, C., et al. "Enzyme activity and fiber composition in skeletal muscle of untrained and trained men." *J Appl Physiol* 33:312-319, 1972.
8. Komi, P., Rusko, H., Vos, J., et al. "Anaerobic performance capacity in athletes." *Acta Physiol Scand* 100:107-114, 1977.
9. Lamb, D.R. *Physiology of Exercise: Responses & Adaptations*, 2nd Ed. New York, NY: Macmillan, 1984.
10. Magel, J., Andersen, K.L. "Pulmonary diffusing capacity and cardiac output in young trained Norwegian swimmers and untrained subjects." *Med Sci Sports* 1:131-139, 1969.
11. Skinner, J.S. "Functional effects of physical activity." *In* Zeigler, E.F. (Ed), *Physical Education and Sport: An Introduction*. Philadelphia, PA: Lea & Febiger, 1982.

12. Skinner, J.S., Noeldner, S.P., O'Connor, J.S. "The development and maintenance of physical fitness." *In* Ryan, A.J., Allman, F.D. (Eds), *Sports Medicine*, 2nd Ed. New York, NY: Academic Press, 1989.

13. Thorstensson, A., Larsson, L., Tesch, P., et al. "Muscle strength and fiber composition in athletes and sedentary men." *Med Sci Sports* 9:26-30, 1977.

14. Wilmore, J.H., Costill, D.L. *Training for Sport and Activity*, Ed 3. Dubuque, IA: Wm. C. Brown Publishers, 1988.

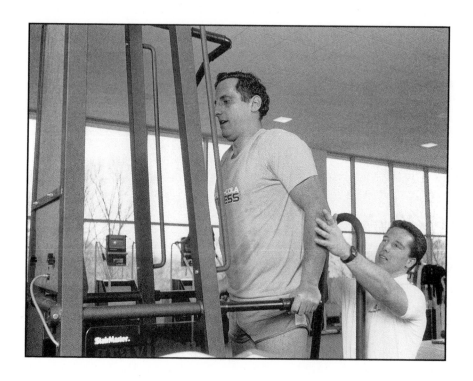

CHAPTER 5

• •

UNDERSTANDING THE PHYSIOLOGICAL BASIS OF MUSCULAR FITNESS

by

James E. Graves, Ph.D.
and
Michael L. Pollock, Ph.D.

• • •

Muscular fitness is one of the primary parameters of physical fitness. It involves two basic components: muscular strength[1] and muscular endurance.[2] It is developed by placing a demand (overload) on the muscles of an individual. As the individual's body adapts to the demand, the individual becomes stronger or better able to sustain muscular activity, depending on the nature of the demand.

The process of overloading the muscular system is commonly referred to as resistance training.[3] Resistance training not only can develop muscular strength and muscular endurance, it can also improve the ability of the muscles to recover more quickly from the stresses imposed by physical activity. In addition, properly performed resistance training has been found to produce an increase in an individual's level of muscle mass, bone mineral density, and strength of connective tissue. All of these changes have been shown to have a positive effect on fitness and health—particularly as an individual ages.

Research has documented the fact that physical fitness declines with age. However, many of the detrimental age-related changes in physiological function

---

[1] Muscular strength refers to the ability to generate force at a given speed (velocity) of movement (Knuttgen and Kraemer, 1987).

[2] Muscular endurance refers to the ability to persist in physical activity or resist muscular fatigue (Baumgartner and Jackson, 1987).

[3] The term "resistance" training is used in this chapter to cover all types of "strength" or "weight" training including free weight, isokinetic, variable resistance, and isometric.

are due to decreased physical activity associated with aging and can be attenuated or even reversed with proper exercise training. Just as aerobic training is required for the development and maintenance of cardiorespiratory fitness, resistance training is required for the development and maintenance of muscular fitness.

The importance of resistance training for maintaining muscle mass was recently illustrated in a study of master athletes. The investigators measured the aerobic capacity and body composition of 24 master track athletes, 50 to 82 years of age, over a ten-year period. The results showed that when aerobic training was maintained, cardiorespiratory fitness remained unchanged over the course of the study. Percent body fat, however, increased significantly—even among those athletes who maintained their aerobic training. The change in percent fat was attributed to a reduction in fat-free weight (muscle mass), specifically in the upper body, and not an increase in fat weight. Three athletes who supplemented their aerobic training with either resistance training or cross-country skiing, were able to maintain their upper body muscle mass.

In recognition of the need for a well-rounded training program to develop and maintain muscular as well as cardiorespiratory fitness, the American College of Sports Medicine (ACSM) recently revised its original Position Stand on "The Recommended Quantity and Quality of Exercise for Developing and Maintaining Fitness in Healthy Adults" to include a resistance training component. The ACSM recommends resistance training of a moderate- to high-intensity, sufficient to develop and maintain muscle mass, as an integral part of an adult fitness program. One set of 8-12 repetitions of eight to ten exercises that conditions the major muscle groups at least two days per week is the recommended minimum.

In addition to the development and maintenance of muscular strength and muscle mass, the physiological benefits of resistance training include increases in bone mass and in the strength of connective tissue. These adaptations are beneficial for middle-aged and older adults, and in particular postmenopausal women who rapidly lose bone mineral density. Research has also shown that the following additional health benefits[4] are associated with resistance training:

- Modest improvements in cardiorespiratory fitness
- Reductions in body fat
- Modest reductions in blood pressure
- Improved level of glucose tolerance
- Improved blood lipid-lipoprotein profiles

Muscular fitness is required for successful performance in many sports. Thus, resistance training is common among recreational and professional athletes who wish to enhance athletic performance. Resistance training is also prescribed in rehabilitation programs designed to facilitate recovery from accidents and

---

[4] These health benefits have been most often associated with circuit weight training, a method of resistance training in which a series of exercises are performed in succession with only a minimal amount of rest allowed between exercises.

sport-related injuries. The effectiveness of resistance-training exercises in clinical rehabilitation is well documented.

An important benefit associated with resistance training is to reduce the risk of orthopedic injury. Strong muscles support and, thus, help protect the joints that they cross. It is also recognized that inadequate muscular strength can lead to serious musculoskeletal disorders that result in pain and discomfort and loss of income due to disability and premature retirement. The overall strengthening of the musculoskeletal system (muscle, bone and connective tissue) resulting from resistance training has been shown to reduce the risk of elbow and shoulder injuries in tennis players and swimmers. Resistance training may have an even greater importance for individuals participating in contact sports and in reducing the risk of injury due to accidents. Low back pain is a major medical problem in our society. Increasing muscular strength may reduce the risk of developing low back pain as well as reduce the symptoms of pain in low back pain patients. Thus, the adaptations to resistance training increase the potential for a greater quality of life. This chapter will address the basic physiological adaptations to resistance training and methods of assessing muscular fitness.

PHYSIOLOGICAL ADAPTATION TO RESISTANCE TRAINING

NEURAL ADAPTATIONS

It was once believed that the ability of a muscle to generate force depended solely on the size of the muscle: as muscles increased in size (hypertrophy) they became stronger, and as they decreased in size (atrophy), they became weaker. It is now known that muscular strength is determined not only by the size of the muscles, but also by the ability of the nervous system to activate the muscles. In fact, there are a number of short-term resistance training studies that have demonstrated increases in muscular strength with no accompanying hypertrophy.

Skeletal muscles are innervated by motor neurons. Groups of individual muscle fibers that are innervated by the same motor neuron are called motor units. The amount of force generated during muscle contraction depends on two factors: the number of motor units that are fired and the frequency of motor unit firing. Firing frequency refers to the rate of firing or the number of nerve impulses per unit of time that the motor unit receives.

Neural adaptations to resistance training include both an increase in the number of motor units that can be fired at any given time and an increase in the frequency of motor unit firing. Increasing the number of motor units that are fired at a given time may be caused by an increase in the neural drive to the muscle and/or a removal of neural inhibition. Improved coordination among agonist muscles (muscles that work together to produce a specific movement) and removal of activation of antagonist muscles (muscles that produce force and movement in the opposite direction) may also contribute to an increased ability to generate greater muscular force following resistance training.

In young subjects, neural adaptations to resistance training predominate during the first four weeks of a training program, while morphological changes (hypertrophy) to the muscle itself predominate thereafter. In older subjects, neural adaptations are the primary mechanism for increased strength for a period of at least eight weeks. Because most studies typically involve training programs that last 8 to 20 weeks, much of the documented improvements in muscle strength are related to a combination of neural and morphological adaptations. There is relatively little information available on the specific mechanisms of muscular strength gains found during long-term training.

MORPHOLOGICAL ADAPTATIONS

An increase in muscle size is probably the most readily recognized adaptation to resistance training. Such an increase is often observed following as little as two months training. Two theories (hypertrophy vs. hyperplasia) have been advanced to explain the phenomenon of increased muscle size in response to overload stress. The majority of research supports the notion that greater muscle size results from the enlargement (hypertrophy), not proliferation (hyperplasia), of individual muscle fibers. Support for the hyperplasia hypothesis in humans comes from studies of certain athletes (e.g., swimmers, kayakers, body builders) who display hypertrophy of specific muscles even though fiber diameters are relatively small. It is unknown from these cross-sectional studies, however, how many fibers were present prior to training.

Studies on laboratory animals indicate that the number of muscle fibers is genetically determined. In addition, in order for hyperplasia to be an adaptive phenomenon the new fibers would have to become completely separate from the existing fibers and innervated. Such a situation has not been documented. Therefore, the general consensus is that the number of muscle fibers does not increase during postnatal growth and under normal training conditions, hyperplasia does not occur in humans.

The degree of skeletal muscle hypertrophy induced by resistance training depends on a number of factors which include the characteristics of the training program as well as the potential for the muscle to increase in size. Human skeletal muscle is made up of two distinct fiber types: Type I or slow-twitch (oxidative) fibers which have a high capacity for aerobic or endurance types of activities, and Type II or fast-twitch (glycolytic) fibers which are best suited for activities that require strength, speed, and power. Progressive heavy resistance training stimulates an increase in the cross-sectional area of both Type I and Type II muscle fibers although a greater degree of hypertrophy generally occurs in Type II fibers. The greater degree of hypertrophy found in Type II fibers is probably reflective of a greater involvement of these fibers with resistance training. Likewise, atrophy resulting from disuse occurs to the greatest extent in Type II fibers. There are no studies to indicate that resistance training increases the number of Type II fibers relative to Type I. Therefore, the potential for individuals to increase muscle size and muscle strength may be genetically predetermined by the number of Type II fibers they possess.

The increased cross-sectional area of muscle fibers is associated with an increase in the contractile proteins actin and myosin. The amount of protein in the muscle can increase by increasing protein production (synthesis) or by decreasing the rate at which proteins are broken down. Hypertrophy of Type II fibers occurs primarily through an increase in protein synthesis. Hypertrophy of Type I fibers occurs primarily through a decrease in protein breakdown.

Actin and myosin are organized within the muscle fiber in cylindrical units called myofibrils. Myofibrils increase in both size and number following resistance training. Increased myofibril cross-sectional area following resistance training results from an addition of actin and myosin filaments to the periphery of the myofibril. Similarly, atrophy following immobilization or disuse is associated with a loss of contractile protein from the periphery of the myofibril. Myofibrils increase in number by splitting into two or more daughter myofibrils.

The specific mechanism by which resistance training stimulates increased protein synthesis is unknown. There are currently two hypotheses which have been developed to explain the mechanism responsible for muscle hypertrophy. One hypothesis suggests that the tension developed during resistance exercise provides a signal that is read by the genetic machinery of the cell which in turn stimulates protein synthesis. This hypothesis is supported by the fact that little or no hypertrophy will occur during resistance training when the intensity is low. The second hypothesis involves the theory of breakdown and repair. It is thought that during each training session part of the muscle is broken down and that the repair process gradually builds the muscle up to a higher level. The breakdown and repair hypothesis is supported by studies that have identified skeletal muscle damage following heavy resistance exercise.

Because heavy resistance training is associated with an increase in fiber size but does not necessarily stimulate capillary or mitochondrial proliferation, capillary and mitochondrial density are often found to decrease. That is, resistance training does not change the capillary to fiber ratio but since the fibers have increased in size with no change in the number of capillaries, the capillary density is reduced. A training regimen consisting of a high number of repetitions with moderate loads, however, may induce capillary proliferation. Body builders who emphasize high repetition training systems have been found to have a greater capillary density than weight lifters (e.g., power lifters) who train with heavy loads and fewer repetitions. Although capillary and mitochondrial density may be reduced following resistance training the activity of enzymes reflecting anaerobic metabolism remains unchanged. In addition, significant increases in resting concentrations of anaerobic energy stores such as muscle glycogen, and the high energy phosphates creatine phosphate and ATP have been observed. These adaptations improve the ability of individuals to continue to perform work with moderate to heavy loads (anaerobic capacity or muscular endurance). The morphological adaptations to heavy resistance training are illustrated in Table 5-1.

Table 5-1. Morphological Adaptations to Heavy Resistance Training.

Muscle Fiber Size	▲
Myofibril size	▲
Myofibril number	▲
Contractile Protein Content	▲
Fiber Type Composition	NC
Capillary Density	▼
Mitochondrial Density	▼
Aerobic Enzyme Content	NC or ▼
Anaerobic Enzyme Content	
Glycolytic	NC
Non-glycolytic	NC
Muscle Glycogen	▲
ATP and CP	▲
Lipid Content	NC
Myoglobin Content	▼
Connective Tissue	
Absolute amount	▲
Strength	▲

ATP = adenosine triphosphate; CP = creatine phosphate; ▲ = increase; ▼ = decrease; NC = no changes

ADAPTATIONS TO BONE AND CONNECTIVE TISSUE

Bone is a dynamic tissue that changes in density and form in response to the stresses placed upon it. Immobilization and weightlessness cause a rapid loss of bone mass. Physical activity, on the other hand, has a positive influence on bone mineral density but the rate of adaptation for bone is much slower than that of muscle. The influence of resistance training on bone is highly dependent on hormonal and nutritional conditions. For example, bone loss is common in estrogen deficient postmenopausal women. Estrogen replacement therapy is effective at minimizing this bone loss but only when a sufficient amount of dietary calcium is available.

Cross-sectional studies have shown that athletes who participate regularly in weight bearing or resistance training activities have greater bone densities than sedentary controls. Certain athletes who participate in unilateral sports (e.g., tennis and baseball players) exhibit bone hypertrophy in their dominant (playing) arm. The location and degree of hypertrophy are influenced to a great extent by the specific sport; for example, femur and spine bone density are highest in weight lifters and lowest in swimmers.

Although it is widely recognized that weight-bearing activities can increase bone mineral density, there are relatively few longitudinal studies involving resistance training. Conflicting results exist for the few longitudinal studies conducted on the influence of resistance training on bone density. Much of the discrepancy among results from different studies may be due to issues related to specificity of training and the length of training. It is quite evident that additional research is needed.

Connective tissue has an important role during exercise because it provides the basic structural framework and force conveying network for human movement. Most studies on the influence of exercise on connective tissue have used short term aerobic protocols on animal models. There are relatively few studies that have addressed the effects of resistance training on connective tissues.

Resistance training increases the maximum tensile strength of both tendons and ligaments. Strengthening connective tissue may reduce the likelihood of strains, sprains and other injuries associated with physical activity. Body builders have been found to have similar volume densities for collagen and other non-contractile tissue when compared to untrained controls. This finding suggests that the absolute amount of connective tissue within the muscle increases but because muscle cell size also increases, the proportion of muscle that is made up of connective tissue does not change. Thus, training induced increases in muscle fiber size are accompanied by corresponding increases in connective tissue.

The morphological adaptations to resistance training, as discussed in this section, include increases in the strength and mass of muscle, bone, and connective tissue. These adaptations reduce the risk of orthopaedic injury. While muscular strength can improve rather rapidly through neural mechanisms, noticeable changes to bone and connective tissue take longer to occur.

SPECIFICITY OF TRAINING

Strength increases resulting from resistance training are specific to the type of contraction used in training, the range-of-motion (ROM) through which training occurs, the velocity of contraction during training, and whether exercises are performed unilaterally or bilaterally. These examples of specificity of training are all at least partially attributed to neural adaptation; however, for specificity of contraction type and velocity of contraction there is evidence to suggest that resistance training also has specific effects on the contractile properties of the muscle. Each of these examples of specificity of resistance training will be briefly discussed.

There are two basic types of muscle activity: static and dynamic. In a static (commonly referred to as isometric) contraction the muscle attempts to shorten against a fixed or immovable resistance. Thus, there is no movement of the skeleton and the muscle neither shortens nor is forcibly lengthened. A dynamic contraction involves movement and can be either concentric where the force produced by the muscle is sufficient to overcome the resistance and shortening of the muscle occurs, or eccentric where the muscle exerts force, lengthens, and is overcome by the resistance.

Training a muscle group with dynamic actions (e.g., lifting weights) produces relatively large increases in dynamic muscle strength but only small increases in isometric contraction strength. Isometric training on the other hand, has been shown to improve isometric strength more so than dynamic strength. Studies from our laboratory, however, have shown similar improvements in isometric strength through a full ROM following both isometric and dynamic training when the dynamic training involved slow controlled repetitions through a full ROM. In addition to specificity involving isometric and dynamic modes of training, lifting weights has been shown to improve weight lifting strength to a greater extent than isokinetic (constant velocity) concentric contraction strength.

Increases in voluntary strength are specific to the ROM that is trained for both isometric and dynamic resistance training. A significant transfer of isometric strength within 20° of the training angle occurs following an isometric strength training program. At positions beyond 20° from the training angle, little transfer of isometric strength tends to occur. Thus, when isometric exercises are used to improve muscular strength, training should occur at multiple positions throughout the ROM. When training consists of dynamic muscle actions performed through a limited ROM, strength gains have been noted up to 50° away from the ROM used for training. However, improvements in the untrained ROM have been significantly less than those in the ROM in which training was conducted.

Strength training at slow speeds results in relatively large increases in the ability of the muscle to generate force at slow speeds but relatively small increases during contractions at faster speeds. Training at fast speeds results in specifically larger increases in strength at faster speeds. The carry-over of strength from high speed training to slow speed testing is somewhat greater than the carry-over from slow speed training to fast speed testing. However, it is not clear how much of an influence measurement (impact) artifact[5] associated with isokinetic testing has on these particular findings related to the speed of training.

REDUCED TRAINING

When resistance training programs are terminated, muscular strength and muscle mass can be rapidly lost. An important question related to long-term maintenance of muscular fitness is how much resistance training is required to retain strength. Can people reduce training frequency periodically and still maintain strength? Individuals participating in strength training programs must occasionally reduce or stop training for brief periods of time. Studies on endurance exercise suggest that aerobic capacity can be maintained during reduced training frequency and duration as long as intensity is maintained.

Results from a study conducted at our laboratory indicate that as long as training intensity is maintained, people can reduce training frequency to as little

---

[5] On an isokinetic dynamometer which provides a written recording of force output, an impact artifact is the initial spike that occurs during the concentric movement. This artifact (spike) does not correspond to force production by the muscle; rather, it represents the effect of the accelerating limb engaging the movement arm of the machine.

as one day per week for up to 12 weeks without a significant loss in strength. It may be important to note that the subjects in this reduced training study were initially untrained and had only trained from 12 to 18 weeks. Whether highly trained athletes can reduce training frequency to a similar extent or whether reduced training can be carried out for more than 12 weeks without a loss in strength are not known. Available evidences, however, suggest that missing a workout once in a while or having to reduce training frequency because of a busy schedule will not adversely affect muscular fitness. The important consideration is not to stop training altogether.

MEASUREMENT OF MUSCULAR STRENGTH

The primary function of skeletal muscle is to generate force. In most instances, forces generated by skeletal muscles are used to produce movement or for anatomical stabilization. The measurement of muscle force production is used to assess fitness, identify weakness, evaluate progress in rehabilitation programs, and to measure the effectiveness of resistance training. The maximum amount of force that a muscle or group of muscles generate can be measured by a variety of methods: cable tensiometers, dynamometers, strain-gauge devices, one-repetition maximal (1-RM) tests, or computer assisted force and work output determination. Each of these methods will be briefly described.

Regardless of the method chosen to assess muscular strength, certain conditions are required for accurate and reliable measurements of muscle force output. Body position must be stabilized to allow only the desired movement. In the case of measuring muscle force generation during an isometric contraction, the involved joint or joints at which movement would occur must be isolated. An example of the need for stabilization to isolate a specific group of muscles for functional assessment occurs during the measurement of lumbar extensor torque production. The lumbar extensors work in conjunction with the larger, more powerful, gluteus and hamstring muscles to extend the trunk. If the pelvis is free to move during lumbar extension, the pelvis will rotate as the gluteus and hamstring muscles contract. Pelvic rotation would then contribute to the observed torque. Thus, pelvic stabilization is required to accurately assess isolated lumbar extensor function.

Muscle force production varies through a ROM. The most descriptive measures of muscle function account for this fact. The term "strength curve" is used to describe a plot of the resultant force exerted versus an appropriate measure of the joint configuration. Because of acceleration at the beginning and deceleration at the end of all human movements, and the fact that dynamic strength is influenced by the speed of movement, dynamic strength tests are not appropriate for the quantification of muscle function through a ROM. In addition, if dynamic muscle actions are performed at fast speeds, kinetic forces may be recorded that give an inaccurate measure of true force production. Depending upon the specific exercise movement, these kinetic forces can be potentially dangerous, especially for orthopedic patient populations because of the impact that occurs upon rapid deceleration. In our laboratory at the University of Florida, we have observed that isometric tests can safely and accurately quantify muscle force production through a ROM if multiple joint angles are measured.

A final consideration required for the accurate assessment of muscle force production is whether the mass of the involved body part will influence the measurement. For example, if the force generated by the quadriceps muscles during knee extension does not equal or exceed the mass of the lower leg, no measurable force would be observed. Thus, the mass of the lower leg detracts from observed force production of the quadriceps muscles during knee extension testing. This mass must be accounted for to accurately quantify force. Although there is some controversy concerning the need for correction of the influence of gravitational forces during testing because most bodily activities are not "corrected" for gravity, the actual force generated by specific muscles in certain positions may be greatly influenced by body mass. Thus, although one cannot neglect the fact that in normal daily activities muscles are influenced by body mass, standardization of the testing position and correction for gravitational forces are required for the accurate quantification of muscle force production. The need for stabilization, positional standardization, compensation for gravitational influences and measurement through a ROM have been recently discussed by Pollock et al. (in press).

MEASUREMENT DEVICES

The cable tensiometer is an instrument used to measure static strength by recording the tension applied to a steel cable. This instrument was originally designed to measure aircraft cable tension and was adapted and later refined to measure the strength of various muscle groups. One end of the cable is attached to a fixed object (e.g., a wall or the floor) and the other end is fitted with a bar, a handle, an ankle cuff, or some similar device to which force can be applied by a limb segment. In order for the measurement to accurately reflect muscle force production, the cable must be in the plane of movement and must make a 90° angle at its point of attachment to the body or body part. The tensiometer, which is placed along the length of the cable, measures cable tension when the subject applies force to the cable.

Because the force generating capacity varies through a ROM, establishing the proper angle of measurement is critical. A goniometer is usually used to set the joint angle for testing. The cable tensiometer strength test can accurately measure the static strength of virtually all major muscle groups. The device is highly reliable when used on normal subjects. However, the cable and attachments often stretch during testing which makes positional standardization difficult.

The dynamometer is an instrument used to measure static strength by recording the amount of force exerted. Two portable types of dynamometers are widely available—one for hand grip and one for back and leg strength. The most common type is the hand or grip dynamometer. Grip strength is measured as kilograms of force exerted by squeezing the hand dynamometer as hard as possible.

Portable dynamometers are popular for testing large numbers of people because they are easy to use and portable. Cumbersome set-up procedures that often accompany other types of muscle performance measurements are not necessary. Limitations of dynamometers include the fact that they can be used to measure only a few muscle groups and their reliability is not well established. In addition, isolation of specific muscle groups is not accomplished which makes standardization difficult.

Strain-gauge devices can be employed to measure static and dynamic muscle force capacity for a variety of muscle groups. Strain gauges are made of electroconductive material that is usually applied to the surfaces of finely machined metal parts. When a load (from a muscle contraction) is placed on the metal parts, the metal and the strain gauge attached to it deforms. The deformation of the strain gauge causes change in the electrical resistance of the gauge to a voltage or current passed through it. The change in voltage is related to the load and can be recorded on a strip chart, digital display, or volt meter. In most instances strain-gauges are used to measure static strain or compression by pushing or pulling on the device. Applications of strain gauges for dynamic strength measures, however, are commercially available (e.g., isokinetic machines). Strain gauge measurements are reliable but they have the same limitations as the cable tensiometer.

One-repetition maximum tests measure the greatest amount of weight that can be lifted one time for a specific weight-lifting exercise. These tests are usually limited to the amount of weight that can be lifted at the weakest position in the ROM and, therefore, do not assess muscle performance through a full ROM. Generally the test begins with an amount of weight that can be easily lifted. After a successful trial, a two to three minute rest period is allowed. Then the weight is increased by five to ten pounds (or more depending on the difficulty of the previous lift) and another trial is attempted. The 1-RM is the amount of weight for the last trial that can be successfully completed with good form and can usually be obtained in four to six trials. The 1-RM provides a measure of dynamic strength that can be applied to almost any weight lifting exercise. One repetition maximum tests are popular because they are easy to administer and can often be performed with the same equipment used for training. They are highly reliable although they do involve a factor of skill and subsequent tests may yield greater results due to practice. Thus, 1-RM tests may not be specific for muscle force production.

The application of computer technology and advancements in machine design have improved the accuracy and standardization of muscular strength testing. Electromechanical dynamometers have been developed for both static and dynamic measures of muscular strength. Some electromechanical dynamometers are capable of both static and dynamic strength measurements. Many electromechanical dynamometers employ a load cell to measure static strength. This method may be considered the electronic equivalent of the cable tensiometer. A major advantage of machines that use load cells, however, is the ease of making multiple measurements through a ROM. Cable tensiometer systems are usually cumbersome to adjust and, therefore, are usually used to provide a measure of static strength at only a single joint angle. Because strength varies through a ROM based upon the biomechanical arrangement of the muscles and bony levers of the skeletal system, single joint angle measures do not provide an indication of how strength varies through the ROM. Multiple joint-angle isometric tests are often employed to quantify full ROM static strength. Multiple joint-angle isometric tests have been shown to be highly reliable for a variety of muscle groups.

Some electromechanical instruments have been designed to measure dynamic muscular strength at a pre-set movement speed. In theory, these constant-velocity (isokinetic) dynamometers are thought to measure the maximum force that can be applied throughout the constant velocity movement. Because a period of acceleration is required to reach the pre-selected velocity of movement, and a period of deceleration is required at the end of the movement, isokinetic dynamometers cannot measure force production through a full ROM. In addition, oscillation in observed forces, called torque overshoot, can limit the accuracy of these devices. These torque overshoots represent impact forces between the moving body part and the measurement device. Manufacturers have attempted to overcome these measurement errors by various software controlled averaging systems (called dampening mechanisms) with limited success. While data averaging may be effective at presenting smooth force curves, it cannot eliminate potentially dangerous impact forces. Measurement error associated with isokinetic dynamometry has been discussed in detail. Unfortunately, in spite of their shortcomings, isokinetic dynamometers are a common method of strength assessment in many clinical and research settings.

MEASUREMENT OF MUSCULAR ENDURANCE

Almost all of the devices for measuring strength can also be used for assessing muscular endurance. Tests of muscular endurance should be designed to evaluate the ability of a muscle group to produce submaximal force for an extended duration. More specifically, the length of time a muscle contraction can be held or the number of repeated submaximal contractions a muscle group can make should be determined. Accordingly, similar to strength, muscular endurance can be assessed either statically or dynamically.

MEASURING MUSCLE ENDURANCE STATICALLY

Two basic methods exist for assessing muscular endurance statically. One method involves having an individual perform a maximal static contraction and sustain that level of contraction for 60 seconds. The force being exerted by the muscle should be recorded at 10-second intervals. Accordingly, individuals who experience a slower rate of decline in force production are exhibiting a greater level of muscle endurance for that specific muscle group than those whose level of recorded force falls at a faster rate. The other method for statically assessing muscular endurance is to determine how long a given percentage of an individual's maximum voluntary contraction (MVC) strength can be sustained.

MEASURING MUSCLE ENDURANCE DYNAMICALLY

A number of ways exist for determining muscular endurance dynamically. One way dynamic muscle endurance can be assessed is for an individual to perform the maximum number of repetitions possible using an absolute weight, a given percentage of maximum strength, or some set percentage of body weight. The endurance of a muscle group can be determined isokinetically through the performance of successive maximal repetitions. Isokinetic muscular endurance is measured as the number of repetitions completed before the torque production drops below 50% of the maximal torque value. Perhaps the most commonly used method for evaluating muscular endurance is calisthenic-type (e.g., sit-ups, push-ups, pull-ups, etc.) exercise testing. During such tests, the maximum number of times an individual can lift his or her own body weight is used as the measure of endurance. For individuals of below-average muscular fitness or above-average body weight, however, calisthenic-type exercises can often involve more of a measure of muscular strength than muscular endurance. ❏

BIBLIOGRAPHY •

1. American College of Sports Medicine. "Position stand: The recommended quantity and quality of exercise for developing and maintaining cardiorespiratory and muscular fitness in healthy adults." *Med Sci Sports Exerc* 22:265-274, 1990.
2. Baumgartner, T.A., Jackson, A.S. *Measurement for Evaluation in Physical Education and Exercise Science.* Dubuque, IA: Wm. C. Brown Publishers, 1987.
3. Fleck, S.J., Kraemer, W.J. *Designing Resistance Training Programs.* Champaign, IL: Human Kinetics Publishers, 1987.
4. Graves, J.E., Pollock, M.L., Carpenter, D.M., et al. "Quantitative assessment of full range-of-motion isometric lumbar extension strength." *Spine* 15(4):289-294, 1990a.
5. Graves, J.E., Pollock, M.L., Foster, D., et al. "Effect of training frequency and specificity on isometric lumbar extension strength." *Spine* 15(6):504-509, 1990b.
6. Graves, J.E., Pollock, M.L., Jones, A.E., et al. "Specificity of limited range of motion variable resistance training." *Med Sci Sports Exerc* 21(1):84-89, 1989.
7. Graves, J.E., Pollock, M.L., Leggett, S.H., et al. "Effect of reduced training frequency on muscular strength." *Int J Sports Med* 9(5):316-319, 1988.
8. Graves, J.E., Welsch, M., Pollock, M.L. "Exercise training for muscular strength and endurance." *Idea Today* 9(7):33-40, 1991.
9. Grimby, G. "Progressive resistance exercise for injury rehabilitation." *Sports Med* 2:309-315, 1985.
10. Jones, N.L., McCartney, N., McComas, A.J. (Eds). *Human Muscle Power.* Champaign, IL: Human Kinetics Publishers, 1986.
11. Knuttgen, H.G., Kraemer, W.J. "Terminology and measurement in exercise performance." *J Appl Sport Sci Res* 1(1):1-10, 1987.
12. Komi, P.V. (Ed). Strength an*d Power in Sport.* Cambridge, MA: Blackwell Scientific Publications, 1992.
13. MacDougall, J.D., Wenger, H.A., Green, H.J. (Eds). Physiological Testing of the *High-Performance Athlete.* Champaign, IL: Human Kinetics Publishers, 1991.

14. Pollock, M.L., Graves, J.E., Carpenter, D.M., et al. "The lumbar musculature: testing and conditioning for rehabilitation." In Hockshulers, G.R., Colter, H., Carranza, C. (Eds), *Rehabilitation of the Spine: Science and Practice*. New York, NY: Springer-Verlag, (in press).

15. Pollock, M.L., Wilmore, J.H. Exercise in Health and Disease: Evaluation and Prescription for Prevention and Rehabilitation, 2nd Ed. Philadelphia, PA: W. B. Saunders Company, 1990.

16. Risch, S., Norvell, N., Pollock M., et al. "Lumbar strengthening in chronic low back pain patients: Psychological and physiological benefits." *Spine* (in press).

17. Stone, M.H., Fleck, S.J., Triplett, N.T., et al. "Health- and performance-related potential of resistance training." *Sports Med* 11(4):210-231, 1991.

CHAPTER 6

● ●

UNDERSTANDING THE PSYCHOLOGICAL BASIS OF EXERCISE

by

Debra J. Crews, Ph.D.
and
Elizabeth Hart, M.A.

● ● ●

*A*n intrinsic interaction between your mind and your body exists during all daily activities, including exercise. The relationship between psychological state and exercise is cyclical, such that your psychological state prior to exercise can influence your physiological response to exercise and the performance outcome. Similarly, exercise is known to influence your psychological state both during and after exercise. Psychological state is usually defined as the mental and emotional processes at a given point in time. Such a definition involves several factors, including affect, mood, stress reactivity, anxiety, depression, cognitive functioning, self-perception, personality characteristics and addictive behaviors. This chapter is divided into two main parts. The first section discusses the influence of *psychological state on exercise.* The other primary section addresses the effects of *exercise on specific psychological states.*

Over the years, research in this area has generally involved an interdisciplinary approach between psychology and exercise science. As a result, in the past two decades the field of exercise psychology has evolved as an effective force in the effort to obtain more accurate information on the relationship between exercise and the mind-body connection. This chapter presents an overview of several of the important research findings concerning this relationship. The critical information within each main section and sub-section is summarized at the end of each particular segment with a special "points to remember" discussion. Viable mechanisms to explain the reason exercise influences each psychological state are also summarized within each section.

PSYCHOLOGICAL INFLUENCES ON EXERCISE

Your psychological state can have a profound effect on your ability to perform physically. Unfortunately, the importance of your psychological state, as it relates to physical performance, is sometimes ignored. For example, it is highly unlikely that if your fitness is assessed in a structured situation such as an exercise facility, a cardiac rehabilitation program, or a laboratory situation that your present psychological state and how it may influence your test results are taken into account. By the same token, how the effectiveness of a particular training regimen might be influenced by specific psychosocial variables on a given day or over a given period of time is also frequently overlooked.

Three categories of psychosocial variables have been identified which influence either the physiological response to exercise or the exercise performance outcome. All variables are grouped into one of three basic classifications: affect/mood, perceptions, and cognitions.

Affect is defined as a state of mind or body, an emotion or feeling related to an idea or object. It tends to be more of an immediate and intense psychological experience. In contrast, mood is an enduring, less intense emotional state representing a predominant or prevailing feeling.

Perception involves the use of senses, awareness, and comprehension to understand objects, qualities, etc. Hypnosis and personality characteristics are two factors that alter an individual's perception and have been found to influence exercise behavior.

The third category—cognitions—refers to the process of knowing. Examples of variables in this classification include memory, judgment, and perception. Exercisers use specific cognitive strategies at various stages of training to enhance their performance outcome. These strategies, which are commonly referred to as coping techniques, include the use of biofeedback in some cases.

Affect/mood. Research has shown that affect/mood influences both your physiological responses during exercise and your performance outcome. One major study was designed in such a way that the conditions of anger, happiness, sadness, and fear using imagery were compared with conditions of relaxation and control while subjects completed a stepping task. Researchers in this investigation found that heart rate (HR) and systolic blood pressure (SBP) were the main reactors during exercise and that anger, fear, and happiness produced more step climbing in less time compared with the control condition. The HR of subjects in this study actually doubled during the anger and exercise conditions. On the other hand, the sadness and relaxation conditions produced lower performance outcomes than the control condition. Sadness also exhibited an inhibitory effect on the HR and diastolic blood pressure (DBP) responses to exercise.

Researchers in other studies have also discovered that affect/mood influences physiological and performance responses. For example, happiness has been shown to produce greater grip strength responses than sadness. In another study, daily variations in running economy (i.e., the oxygen cost of exercise at a given work load) were found to be highly related to overall mood state—specifically, tension (i.e., running economy decreases as tension increases). This particular response, for example, may affect a cardiac rehabilitation patient in an angry state or a sad state who as a result of this specific affect/mood may experience significantly different HRs during training.

Perception. Noted exercise psychologist, William Morgan, has demonstrated through a series of studies that exercisers working at a constant workload will exhibit varying physiological responses during an altered state of consciousness (i.e., hypnosis). For instance, exercisers who are led to believe that they are lifting a heavier weight than they actually are, or are cycling up a hill when they are on level terrain, will have greater oxygen demands and changes in ventilation, respectively.

Type A behavior, which is separately addressed in a latter section of this chapter, has been associated with a more positive perception of exercise at low-to-moderate intensity work and a more negative affect at high intensity work levels than found among individuals with Type B personalities. This finding suggests that your psychological state prior to exercise can influence your perception of the exercise. Accordingly, many researchers conclude that any physiological information monitored during exercise can be influenced at a subconscious level by the exerciser's pre-existing psychological state. Furthermore, they contend that this physiological information is somehow altered prior to reaching the conscious level of awareness in the cerebral cortex of the brain. As a result, these researchers assert that it is highly likely that it is important for an exerciser to attain a positive psychological state prior to exercising in order to receive the greatest benefit from the exercise bout.

In addition to considering the effects of psychological factors on exercise, it is also important to note the effect of exercise on your perception of the exercise as well. The most common measure of perceived effort during exercise is the rating of perceived exertion (RPE). Exertion or RPE has been defined by several exercise scientists as the integration of various *physiological* sensations. A strong argument could be advanced that RPE would be more appropriately defined as the integration of various *psychosocial* influences and *physiological* sensations. RPE, using this definition, would involve both physiological cues (two-thirds) and psychological cues (one-third). Psychological cues are believed to have a greater influence during low and moderate intensity exercise, while physiological cues dominate RPE assessment at high-intensity work levels. Among the various psychosocial factors which are associated with a decrease in RPE are: extroversion, hypnosis, dissociation, anxiety, gender of the exercise tester, and athletic experience.

RPE was originally structured to provide scores which were almost linearly related to HR (RPE x 10 = HR). In a few studies, however, ventilation and lactate levels have been found to have a closer relationship with RPE scores than HR. Such findings suggest that some degree of caution is necessary when you're using

RPE to determine training intensity. The intensity of the exercise bout should be assessed by at least one additional physiological measure, as well as through the use of RPE, since several psychological factors have been shown to influence RPE.

Cognition. The three categories within cognition which have been shown to influence exercise include: mental strategies (e.g., association, dissociation), coping strategies (e.g., stress management, relaxation), and biofeedback (information provided to an individual regarding a physiological response during exercise).

The two mental strategies which have received the greatest attention are association and dissociation. Association refers to an attentional focus on bodily responses during exercise. In contrast, dissociation refers to an attentional focus on anything other than bodily responses. It appears that beginning exercisers benefit most from dissociative techniques. Advanced exercisers encounter a similar experience when they participate in a novel task. Novice exercisers seem to benefit most from distraction, or dissociation, since they are not familiar with the pain or discomforts of starting an exercise program, and, thus, have not devised appropriate coping strategies for dealing with the pain.

Experienced exercisers participating in an exercise mode familiar to them benefit most from an associative style. Individuals who exercise on a regular basis in a familiar activity learn the (coping) techniques necessary for controlling their pain and discomfort. Focusing on bodily responses during exercise evokes the cues needed for eliciting the appropriate coping technique. It is important to note, however, that during an exercise bout, you use both associative and dissociative strategies, and that your adherence to one strategy does not usually exceed 80% of the total time you exercise. Exercise psychologists caution exercisers to keep in mind the fact that the existing research suggests that these two mental strategies do not adequately encompass all of the thoughts you use to control your responses while exercising. Unfortunately, however, they conclude that until which time more precise definitions and conclusive classifications are identified and tested, these two strategies offer the best basis for explaining how you cognitively attempt to influence your response to exercise.

Stress management is probably the coping strategy most commonly used during exercise. Stress management includes relaxation, visualization, imagery, biofeedback, and cognitive restructuring (e.g., changing self-talk patterns). Research has shown that oxygen cost decreases during the first half of an aerobic exercise bout for individuals who employ stress management techniques. Other studies have found that the use of relaxation techniques has resulted in enhanced running performance. Researchers conclude that such performance changes are probably the consequence of improvements in running economy which result from the reduction in the tension level experienced by the exercisers.

Several biofeedback studies have examined the effects of manipulating a specific physiological response during exercise to determine what changes occur in the energy cost of exercise or in the performance outcome. Recent research suggests, however, that such studies have substantial methodological limitations. The majority of these studies, for example, have used a single physiological response measure to alter the cost or the performance result of an exercise bout. The use of multiple physiological measures, however, has been found to be more effective in producing changes in exercise economy and performance. Studies employing multiple physiological measures have shown that programs using biofeedback may have to be conducted over a relatively longer period of time to produce substantial changes in the energy cost levels of the exercisers. Furthermore, researchers surmise that any changes in the performance outcome of an exercise bout are likely to be subsequent to changes in energy economy levels.

POINTS TO REMEMBER

- Anger, fear, and happiness produce greater physiological responses during exercise and better performance outcomes, while sadness inhibits these responses.
- Anxiety has been shown to increase the energy cost of exercise on a given day.
- Your psychological state prior to exercise can influence the ratings of effort you experience during exercise.
- RPE should be used in conjunction with a physiological measure since many psychological factors influence RPE.
- Novice exercisers effectively use dissociative strategies, while experienced exercisers effectively use associative strategies while exercising on a mode familiar to them.
- Stress management techniques can reduce the oxygen cost of exercise.
- Biofeedback training can effectively alter a physiological response pattern. Multimeasure biofeedback training, however, appears to be the most effective way to reduce the oxygen cost of exercise and ultimately, to improve performance.

THE EFFECTS OF EXERCISE ON SPECIFIC PSYCHOLOGICAL STATES

Among the many benefits often attributed to exercise is the perception that exercise improves your ability to perform certain tasks and to think more clearly. In fact, many corporations, for example, have made substantial investments in exercise facilities at least partially on the belief that their employees who use these facilities will be, not only healthier, but more productive as a result of the opportunity to exercise on a regular basis. The possible effect of exercising on cognitive functioning gives rise to several questions. First, do individuals think better or perform tasks more efficiently if they exercise on a regular basis? More specifically, does their cognitive functioning improve during and/or after exercise? At least two factors should be considered when attempting to answer this question. First, what type of exercise influences cognitive functioning? Second, what aspects of performance are influenced by exercise?

Research findings suggest that exercise does influence cognitive functioning. How it affects your ability to think and perform certain tasks appears to depend on certain features attendant to the general type of exercise in which you engage—for example, how often and how long you exercise. Acute (e.g., a single exercise bout) exercise, for example, differs widely from chronic (e.g., repeated exercise bouts over time) exercise in the way it affects cognitive functioning. When examining cognitive performance during or immediately after exercise, it appears that an exercise bout of high intensity and short duration enhances performance. In addition, as the intensity of an exercise bout is reduced, its duration may be lengthened (within limits) without incurring a concomitant decrement in performance. On the other hand, exercising a relatively longer period of time that produces fatigue has been shown to have a debilitating effect on cognitive performance. Tasks involving speed rather than accuracy have been shown to be enhanced by an acute bout of exercise. Moderate difficulty tasks are most likely to improve with exercise rather than tasks which are at either end of the spectrum (e.g., too easy or too difficult).

Chronic exercise has been associated, both during and following physical activity, with levels of higher intelligence and enhanced memory. It is not clear whether intelligent people choose to exercise or whether exercise affects intelligence. It also appears that exercise enhances memory recall. Such a finding has very important implications—particularly for older populations.

The mechanism by which exercise may influence cognitive functioning has received considerable attention by researchers. One theory which has been advanced suggests that increases in core temperature, which accompany exercise, may speed specific catalytic events in the body which facilitate cognitive functioning and performance. Core temperatures, for example, may be elevated for as long as 90 minutes after you stop exercising. Credence to this theory has been provided by investigators who have been able to show that exercise in which core temperature changes are blocked inhibits improvements in cognitive performance via altered brain wave patterns. Another possible explanation for the relationship between exercise and cognitive functioning has been termed by researchers as the "hardware" alteration. This interpretation suggests that the density of blood vessels in your cerebral cortex increases as the result of exercise, while the number of synapses associated with a particular motor activity increases as you learn the activity. The temperature and the structural changes interact with each other in such a way to produce improved cognitive functioning.

POINTS TO REMEMBER
- Short duration, high intensity exercise facilitates cognitive functioning (specifically speed), both during and after exercise.
- Exercise of a moderate duration and a moderate intensity also facilitates cognitive performance both during and after exercise. The effects are larger for moderate difficulty tasks.
- Longer duration, low intensity exercise enhances your ability to think clearly and perform certain motor functions until you become fatigued. Fatigue inhibits cognitive functioning and performance.

EXERCISE INFLUENCES ON STRESS REACTIVITY

Many individuals who lead an active lifestyle often believe that exercise reduces the stresses which arise during daily living. Stress is an emotional response which occurs when the demands of a situation exceed an individual's perceived capabilities to handle that situation in an appropriate manner. What these exercisers may be perceiving is that exercise reduces the extent of their response to the self-defined stressors in their life. As a result, they subsequently spend less time in a "stressful" state. The potential impact of such a consequence can be significant. For example, some evidence exists to support the contention that decreasing the extent and the time for which you are suffering from stress elicits a concomitant reduction in your level of cardiovascular risk and improves your immunological competence (e.g., your resistance to infection and disease).

The basic assumption by which exercise is believed to have a positive effect on stress suggests that your physiological response to exercise is somewhat similar to your physiological response during stress. Accordingly, exercise may train your body to more effectively cope with the daily stressors you encounter. On the other hand, a few subtle differences exist between your physiological response to exercise as compared to psychological stress. One of the more obvious differences lies in the source of where in your body the physiological response is initiated. On one hand, the demands of exercise elicit increases in primarily sympathetic activation from the periphery of your body (e.g., your muscles). On the other hand, your response to psychological stress is initiated from the central command center of your brain. The common factor in your physiological reaction to both exercise and psychological stress is the response of your adrenal system. Research findings in this area suggest that your adrenal receptor sensitivity is altered by exercise, thus reducing your physiological response to stress.

Despite the subtle differences which exist between your physiological responses to exercise and stress, the available data indicate that you will experience an overall reduction in your stress level as a result of exercise. Most of the research on this subject has attempted to identify the effect of chronic aerobic exercise on stress reactivity by comparing fit with unfit individuals. Fit subjects have been found to exhibit both a reduced reactivity to stress and an enhanced ability to recover to their pre-stress emotional state following a bout of stress.

Only a limited amount of research has been conducted which has examined the effects of an acute bout of exercise on stress. Unfortunately, these studies have produced equivocal results depending on the amount of time which has elapsed between when an exercise bout occurred and when the stressor was present. For example, a group of researchers from Wake Forest University were able to demonstrate a reduction in HR and SBP reactivity when the subjects were allowed a 30-minute recovery period following their exercise session. In addition, these researchers found that higher intensity exercise produced a greater reduction in HR and SBP response to psychosocial stressors than did low intensity exercise.

Finally, anaerobic exercise should not be ignored as a potential means of reducing stress. At least one group of investigators have reported findings that indicate that anaerobic exercise reduces stress reactivity more effectively than aerobic exercise.

Several theories have been advanced to explain the possible basis regarding why stress reactivity is reduced following exercise. The "time-out hypothesis" suggests that time away from the stressor reduces stress. Yet, this hypothesis does not explain why higher intensity exercise elicits greater reductions in stress reactivity than lower intensity exercise. The "opponent process theory" suggests that the physical stress of exercise may produce an opposing response (e.g., reduced stress) following exercise. Dienstbier's "sympathetic toughness concept" proposes that repeated exposure to physical stress (e.g., exercise) may train your body to be less affected by certain demands on it and recover more quickly from psychosocial stress.

The finding that exercise can have a positive effect on stress reactivity has several potential implications for other health benefits, such as reduced cardiovascular risk and enhanced immunological function. Considerable research has confirmed that your level of stress is a significant causal factor in both coronary heart disease and immune system response. Accordingly, the ability of exercise to decrease your level of stress reactivity can have a corresponding positive influence not only on how well you handle stress, but also on the effect of that stress on your exposure to certain diseases. A lower blood pressure response reduces your level of cardiovascular risk, which subsequently diminishes the likelihood that you will suffer from coronary heart disease. The research findings concerning the possible effect that exercise has on immune function are equally promising. Data is available which show that aerobic exercise has a positive effect on natural killer cell activity, thereby enhancing immunological competence.

POINTS TO REMEMBER
- Acute aerobic exercise with adequate recovery time reduces stress reactivity among conditioned individuals. These effects are greater following high intensity exercise.
- Chronic aerobic exercise reduces both stress response and your ability to recover from stress.
- Anaerobic exercise appears to reduce stress reactivity.
- Exercise which reduces stress may also reduce cardiovascular risk and enhance immunological competence.

EXERCISE INFLUENCES ON ANXIETY, MOOD STATE, AND DEPRESSION

People often report that they "feel better" after exercising. "Feeling better" may represent many responses to exercise, including physiological responses (increased energy), perceptual responses (enhanced self-esteem), and affective responses (reduction of negative thoughts and feelings).

Exercise psychologists are particularly interested in these responses to exercise since they may help to explain individual motives for exercise involvement and adherence. This section of the chapter explores the influence of exercise on emotion or, as it is more commonly referred to in the exercise literature—"affect." Specifically, the influence of exercise on anxiety, general mood state and depression is addressed.

Anxiety and General Mood State. A recent scientific review of the effects of exercise on anxiety and mood combined the results from a variety of investigations. Researchers involved in this effort concluded that exercising can improve both anxiety and mood over baseline levels. The type of comparison group used, the type of exercise performed, and the intensity and duration of the exercise bout were all found to influence this relationship. For example, some of the investigations compared the effect of an exercising group to a non-exercising group and found that exercise reduced anxiety and improved mood levels. Other studies compared participants to each other before and after exercising and still found that a reduction in anxiety and an improvement in mood levels resulted. Other investigators compared an exercising group to a placebo control group (e.g., yoga, relaxation). In these research efforts, exercise was found to be somewhat better in improving mood state than the placebo control treatment.

The findings of these studies suggest that the effects of exercise on anxiety are dependent on whether the anxiety is short-term ("state anxiety") or more chronic ("trait anxiety"). Exercise does not reduce state anxiety to a greater degree than "other activities." These results lend some support to the "time-out" hypothesis regarding why stress levels are reduced following exercise—a theory which suggests that exercise may serve simply as a distraction from your daily worries.

Long-term exercise appears to reduce trait anxiety to a greater extent than shorter-term exercise. This reduction is commonly linked to the "training" effect that accompanies long-term exercise participation. Many researchers have shown that exercise itself represents a physiological stressor. Accordingly, regular exposure to exercise subsequently reduces your body's negative response to exercise. In turn, after an appropriate period of time, regular exercise elicits specific positive reactions which "toughen" it, thereby enabling it to respond in a more appropriate manner to other subsequent stressors (e.g., physiological and/or psychological).

The duration and intensity of exercise have been found to influence anxiety and mood state. It appears that exercise needs to be performed at least 20 minutes at an intensity of greater than 70% HR-max to be associated with reduced anxiety and improved mood. Exercise bouts lasting longer than 30 minutes have not been shown to result in greater changes. Increasing intensities of exercise, however, have been associated with a more positive mood state and reduced anxiety. A few studies have explored anxiety and mood responses to exercise intensities as high as 90%. The findings from these studies indicate that exercising at extremely high intensity levels may have a negative effect on both anxiety and mood state. Reductions in anxiety and mood improvements have been reported to continue for at least 30 minutes, and perhaps as long as six hours, after the exercise bout has actually ceased. The type of exercise performed is yet another factor which appears to influence whether an anxiety reduction or mood state improvement occurs. The majority of the research performed in this area has focused on aerobic exercise—the type of activity which has been shown to have the most positive affect on anxiety and mood state levels. Unfortunately, relatively little is known about the effects of anaerobic exercise on anxiety and mood state.

Exercise Influences on Depression. Exercise has long been advocated as a possible positive factor in the treatment of depression. Early research on the subject suggested that higher levels of depression existed primarily in individuals who exhibited lower levels of fitness. As a result, it was erroneously believed that only poorly fit people could diminish their feelings of depression by exercising and that the general population would not receive a similar benefit. Eventually, however, researchers rightfully concluded that such research had several significant design limitations. For example, information which explained the degree of depression or the type of exercise intervention in the study was frequently not reported in the summary of the research findings.

Recently, many studies have shown that both acute and chronic exercise significantly decrease depression. Contrary to other findings, these results suggest that the antidepressant effect of exercise may begin in the first session of exercise. In addition, these studies have found that exercise is a better antidepressant than relaxation or other "enjoyable" activities, and is as effective in decreasing depression as psychotherapy. It is important to note, however, that considerable evidence exists which indicates that exercise when combined with psychotherapy is a more effective alternative than exercise alone in reducing depression. Finally, decreases in levels of depression have been observed across a variety of subject characteristics, including age, gender, and degree of depression. In terms of reducing depression, exercise has been found to be effective across all age groups, for both men and women, and for varying degrees of depression. Contrary to the earlier assumptions, this finding indicates that exercise will have a positive effect on the level of depression among the general population, not just the deconditioned person.

A variety of explanations have been advanced regarding the antidepressant effects of exercise. The reasons offered generally fall into one of two categories: psychological or physiological. The psychological factors which have been proposed include cognitive-behavioral changes, social interaction factors and the "time-out" hypothesis.

The cognitive changes that may occur as a result of exercise include an increased level of self-confidence and self-esteem that often results when you meet the challenges of a task that you perceive to be somewhat difficult (e.g., exercise). In turn, your ability to master one set of challenges often enables you to be better prepared to deal with different challenges in other areas of your life—all of which may lead to a decrease in your sense of depression.

The belief that social interaction factors can have a positive effect on depression levels implies that contact with others may lead to decreases in depression. Some researchers suggest that the social aspects of exercise may be more influential at the onset of an exercise program, since the rewards of exercise are primarily external and have not been internalized at this point. Such a conclusion, however, was not supported by the findings of a recent study which discovered that exercise programs conducted in the home led to greater decreases in depression than those in either community center or university settings. As was discussed in a previous section in this chapter, the "time-out" hypothesis suggests that exercise may simply offer a distraction from daily worries and problems.

The physiological factors which have been advanced to explain the antidepressant effects of exercise include an increase in cardiovascular fitness, biochemical changes and the release of endorphins. It is highly unlikely, however, that the antidepressant effect of exercise which occurs during the first few weeks of exercise is due to training-induced improvements in cardiovascular fitness (which have not occurred to any substantial extent for most individuals at this particular point in the training regimen). While it is possible that the initial increases in cardiovascular fitness you experience play some role in decreasing chronic depression, the acute effects of exercise may be better explained by the occurrence of specific biochemical alterations in your body. Depressed individuals are thought to have decreased secretions of specific neurotransmitter metabolites which are thought to increase during exercise. As a result, exercise is believed to stimulate the release of these substances, which in turn reduces depression. The release of endorphins (endogenous opiates) are also frequently cited as the mechanism for the alteration of mood state. While increases in endorphin levels have been observed in the blood of humans, they have not been found in the brain. Although euphoric feelings have been linked to endorphin release, until research determines whether endorphins cross the blood-brain barrier, any hypothesis regarding their mood altering properties remains speculation.

POINTS TO REMEMBER
- Exercise needs to be performed for a period lasting at least 20 minutes, at an intensity level of at least 70% HR-max, in order to reduce anxiety and improve mood state.
- Chronic, rather than acute, exercise may be needed to decrease depression.
- Exercise appears to reduce depression in a variety of populations, but the precise mechanism for its antidepressant effect has not, at this point, been identified.

EXERCISE INFLUENCES ON PERSONALITY CHARACTERISTICS

Your personality represents the unique product of your stable and enduring behaviors. In recent years, exercise psychologists have shown an increased interest in exploring the influence that exercise may have on an individual's personality. In particular, individual behaviors that may be related to health risk have received increased attention. The Type A behavior pattern (TABP) is perhaps the most widely studied of these personality characteristics, since it has been linked to coronary heart disease.

The Type A personality is characterized by a strong sense of time urgency, impatience, hostility, aggressiveness, and competitiveness. These characteristics are thought to influence cardiovascular reactivity and neuroendocrine responses, both of which are related to coronary heart disease. It is generally accepted that aerobic exercise lessens cardiovascular reactivity to psychosocial stress. As a result, researchers are interested in the effect that exercise has on Type A individuals, since these individuals often exhibit exaggerated cardiovascular responses to both exercise and stress.

In a recent study which investigated the effect of aerobic exercise on cardiovascular reactivity in Type A middle-aged men, exercise was found to be a promising intervention strategy. In addition, the cardiovascular benefits of aerobic exercise have been found to decrease diastolic blood pressure, heart rate and total peripheral resistance in borderline hypertensive Type A men.

Modifications in the characteristic TABP may also result from engaging in regular exercise. One study found that the basic TABP was modified to a limited extent in Type A females after only 10 weeks of participating in an aerobic exercise program. Some researchers caution, however, that even though some research findings lend support for exercise as a promising intervention in reducing TABP, additional factors must also be considered. First, the majority of Type A intervention research has focused on aerobic exercise. As a result, relatively little is known about the effects of anaerobic exercise. Also, much of the early Type A research utilized a Type A measurement tool (the Jenkins Activity Survey) whose reliability as a predictor of the relationship between TABP and coronary heart disease has recently come into question. In the past few years, the Structured Interview technique has become the preferred assessment tool in this area. The findings of studies using this tool suggest that TABP may not be as directly related to coronary heart disease as was originally thought. Finally, specific components of the Type A personality may be more strongly related to coronary heart disease than the collective (global) measure. In particular, the element of hostility has been identified as one of the personality components most highly linked to coronary heart disease. Interestingly, mood states such as depression and anxiety have been found to be equally valid predictors of coronary heart disease as the collective TABP. Accordingly, a strong argument can be advanced that it may be necessary to reduce specific components of the Type A personality to reduce coronary risk.

POINTS TO REMEMBER

- Aerobic exercise has been shown to change certain aspects of characteristic Type A behaviors.
- Exercise may modify specific components of the TABP that are closely related to coronary heart disease (e.g., hostility) rather than overall TABP.
- The most appropriate way to assess TABP remains an unresolved issue, which raises questions concerning the results from early studies on the effect of exercise on this personality characteristic which used an instrument which has since been somewhat discredited.
- Anxiety and depression have been found to be equally valid predictors of coronary heart disease as the Type A personality characteristic, while hostility may be an even more valid measure.

EXERCISE INFLUENCES ON SELF PERCEPTIONS

A commonly held notion in much of the popular literature suggests that positive perceptions of your body may be related to positive feelings about your self. Given the ingrained nature of this belief, it is quite possible that your self-perceptions may be influenced by your involvement in an exercise program. Early studies conducted in this area reported that participation in exercise programs was associated with improved self-esteem scores. Recent research, however, suggests that self-esteem is a global characteristic that is multidimensional in nature, representing a variety of subcomponents. For example, on one hand, you may have a high degree of esteem specific to your role as a parent; on another hand, you may have a low degree of esteem specific to your body. As a result, it is not all that unlikely that individuals with similar self-esteem scores may differ tremendously on the individual components that collectively comprise their global index of self-esteem.

In addition, the subcomponents of self-esteem may be further divided into more specific dimensions. For example, some researchers suggest that the physical component of self-esteem involves several dimensions. Several researchers have surmised that physical self-esteem is composed of physical self-efficacy, physical competence, and physical acceptance. Others, while also supporting the multidimensional nature of physical self-esteem, propose that physical self-esteem encompasses different factors, including perceptions of sport competence, bodily attractiveness, physical strength and muscular development, and physical conditioning.

When the hierarchical nature of self-esteem is taken into consideration, many exercise psychologists believe that exercise may have more of an immediate effect on the lower levels (specific subcomponents) of self-esteem. In turn, such a consequence has obvious implications regarding how and when physical self-esteem is influenced and, ultimately, global self-esteem. For example, researchers have found that at least 20 weeks of consistent exercise may be needed to observe significant changes in global self-esteem. It appears that the more specific the dimension of self-esteem, the more situationally specific it is in regard to change. Therefore, while participating in an exercise regimen may increase your perceptions of your physical self-attractiveness, it may not have a similar effect on your perception of your sport competence.

Unfortunately, the literature of the relationship between exercise and self-perception is currently somewhat vague and inconclusive. Considerable research does exist, however, to support the contention that the degree of importance an individual places on the physical dimension of self-esteem influences the degree to which exercise participation will influence global self-esteem. In addition, research indicates that factors other than improvements in your level of aerobic fitness may influence the relationship between your exercise participation and your level of physical self-esteem. Changes in your body weight, eating patterns and physical appearance may influence the degree to which your involvement in an exercise program affects your sense of physical self-esteem. Obviously, in this instance, other types of exercise (e.g., resistance training) may also influence particular dimensions of your sense of self-esteem. Attempts to explain the possible influence of exercise on self-esteem have also involved considering whether the sense of accomplishment (that comes when you successfully encounter a challenge) or the opportunity to have positive social interaction with others is consequential.

Finally, research findings indicate that negative physical self-perceptions can also influence whether an individual engages in an exercise program. For example, some individuals will actually avoid exercise (especially in a group setting) if they perceive that others hold a negative opinion of their bodies.

POINTS TO REMEMBER
- The physical self-esteem subcomponent of global self-esteem may be the aspect which is most directly influenced by exercise participation.
- The physical self-esteem subcomponent is divided into specific dimensions which may be differentially affected by various modes of exercise (e.g., running, resistance training).
- The perceived importance you hold for the physical dimension of self-esteem is an important consideration regarding the influence that exercise has on your sense of self-esteem.
- Individuals with a negative opinion regarding the way other individuals will perceive their bodies may avoid participating in physical activities that would otherwise be quite beneficial for them.

EXERCISE AND ADDICTION

Addictive behaviors are often related to poor self-esteem, depression, or high anxiety. Because exercise has been shown to influence these mood states, several efforts have been undertaken in recent years to study exercise as a possible treatment intervention for addictive behaviors. The possible influence of exercising on alcoholism, in particular, has received considerable attention in the past few years. The initial efforts to study the influence of exercise on alcoholism have focused on identifying what physiological changes can be attained by alcoholics who exercise on a regular basis. These studies have attempted to determine whether individuals with a drinking problem could attain improved fitness levels comparable to those achieved by nonalcoholic populations.

A limited amount of research has also attempted to identify the psychological changes in addictive individuals that may result from exercise participation. A reduction in the level of behavioral dysfunction exhibited by these individuals, specifically a decrease in both anxiety and depression, has been reported along with an increase in overall physical fitness. Significant decreases in state anxiety, trait anxiety and depression in alcoholics who exercise on a regular basis have also been observed.

Without question, exercise as a treatment intervention for alcoholism offers some promising findings. Exercise psychologists warn, however, that similar to other research findings in this particular field of specialization, some caution should be taken when interpreting the results of studies involving the possible relationship between exercise and alcoholism. Other alternative explanations should also be considered. For example, participating in an exercise program may enhance the receptivity of an alcoholic to standard psychotherapy intervention. In addition, engaging in a structured leisure-time activity, such as exercise, may cause alcoholics to reorganize the way they spend their leisure time—a process which may in itself serve to discourage past addictive behaviors. Finally, an increased level of fitness may enable an alcoholic to deal more effectively with a specific stress, which, in turn, may reduce the individual's dependence on alcohol.

Interestingly, exercise participation itself may become an addictive behavior. Some researchers suggest that exercise participation should be viewed as a "positive addiction." In other words, the pursuit of the energy and enthusiasm that accompany physical activity is a healthy addiction. Unfortunately, individuals who become dependent on exercise may experience frustration, hostility and guilt when deprived of the opportunity to be physically active. In fact, in one study, the investigators looked at what would happen if individuals were offered money to abstain from exercise for a month. Somewhat surprisingly (depending on your point of view), many habitual exercisers refused to stop participating for the specified length of time regardless of the monetary incentive. Research has also shown that individuals who experience negative feelings when missing a run scored significantly higher on a measure of "commitment to running" than do those who do not. Even short-term variations from running schedules have often been found to have a negative effect on habitual runners.

Researchers have developed the following diagnostic criteria you can review to see if you have a "dependency" on exercise:

- you regularly engage in strenuous exercise (greater than four days per week for at least 30 minutes),

- you suffer from a dysphoric or anxious mood or self-depreciating thoughts when you're unable to exercise as much as planned,
- you alter your normal priorities to the extent that exercise is placed above other activities, with resultant social or occupational consequences,
- you hold irrational expectations regarding the amount of exercise you need to maintain a desired body shape or a perceived level of aerobic fitness,
- you persist with your of exercise behavior in the face of certain negative physical consequences, emanating from such factors as injuries, bad weather or unsafe exercise conditions.

If you recognize a strong similarity between your attitudes and lifestyle and the aforementioned criteria, keep in mind that while exercise may serve as an effective intervention in the treatment of addictive behaviors such as alcoholism, it may become an addictive behavior in your case. In other words, for some, one addiction replaces another. In the initial stages of treatment it may be useful to replace a negative addiction with a positive addiction. Every effort should be made, however, to preclude a positive addiction from being transformed into an addiction with negative consequences.

POINTS TO REMEMBER
- Exercise participation may offer a promising treatment intervention for alcoholism.
- Participation in exercise may enhance an alcoholic's receptivity to standard psychotherapy programs.
- Exercise may offer a positive leisure time activity that replaces past addictive behaviors (e.g., drinking).
- Exercise itself may become addictive leading to abnormal exercise dependence.

THE MIND-BODY CONNECTION

Exercise—particularly aerobic exercise—has been shown to have a positive effect on your state of mind. By the same token, your psychological state has been found to greatly influence what you get out of exercising, including how your body responds physiologically to the demands of the exercise, how much you enjoy the exercise bout, and how your attitudes are shaped regarding the value of exercise (a very component of exercise adherence).

As the field of exercise psychology continues to grow and to expand its efforts to learn more about the mind-body relationship to exercise, the psychological benefits and behavioral consequences of engaging in a sound exercise program will become even more apparent. Eventually, it is not unlikely that exercise prescriptions will address psychological objectives, as well as physiological concerns. Even though exercise psychology is still in its relative infancy, its future is extraordinarily promising. ❏

BIBLIOGRAPHY •

1. Booth-Kewley, S., Friedman, H.S. "Psychological predictors of heart disease: A qualitative review." *Psychol Bull* 101:343-362, 1987.
2. Carmack, M.A., Martens, R. "Measuring commitment to running: A survey of runner's attitudes and mental states." *Sport Psychol* 1:25-42, 1979.
3. Crews, D.J., Landers, D.M. "A meta-analytic review of aerobic fitness and reactivity to psychosocial stressors." *Med Sci Sport Exerc* 19:114-120, 1987.
4. Dientsbier, R.A. "Arousal and physiological toughness: Implications for mental and physical health." *Psychol Rev* 96(1):84-100, 1989.
5. Fiatarone, M.A., Morley, J.E., Bloom, E.T., et al. "Endogenous opioids and the exercise-induced augmentation of natural killer cell activity." *J Lab Clin Med* 112:544-552, 1988.
6. Fox, K.H., Corbin, C.B. "The physical self-perception profile: Development and preliminary validation." *J Sport Exerc Psychol* 11:408-430, 1989.
7. Frankel, A., Murphy, J. "Physical fitness and personality in alcoholism: Canonical analysis of measures before and after treatment." *J Studies Alcohol* 35:1271-1278, 1974.
8. Greist, J.H., Klein, M.H., Eischens, R.R., et al. "Running as a treatment for depression." *Comp Psychiatry* 20:41-54, 1979.
9. Hart, E.A., Leary, M.L., Rejeski, W.J. "The measurement of social physique anxiety." *J Sport Exerc Psychol* 11:94-104, 1989.
10. Kavanagh, D., Hausfeld, S. "Physical performance and self-efficacy under happy and sad moods." *J Sport Psychol* 8:112-123, 1986.
11. Lo, C.R., Phil, D., Johnston, D.W. "The self-control of the cardiovascular response to exercise using feedback of the product of the interbeat interval and pulse transit time." *Psychosom Med* 46:115-125, 1984.
12. Matthews, K.A. "Coronary heart disease and type A behaviors: Update on and alternative to the Booth-Kewley and Friedman (1987) quantitative review." *Psychol Bull* 104:373-380, 1988.
13. Morgan, W.P. "Psychogenic factors and exercise metabolism: A review." *Med Sci Sports Exercise* 17:309-316, 1985.
14. Morgan, W.P., Pollock, M.L. "Psychologic characterizations of the elite distance runner." *Ann NY Acad Sci* 301:382-403, 1977.
15. North, T.C., McCullagh, P., Tran, Z.V. "Effect of exercise on depression." *Exerc Sport Sci Rev* 18:379-415, 1990.
16. Palmer, J., Vacc, N., Epstein, J. "Adult inpatient alcoholics: Physical exercise as a treatment intervention." *J Studies Alcohol* 49(5):418-421, 1988.
17. Pandolf, K.B. "Advances in the study and application of perceived exertion." *Exerc Sport Sci Rev* 11:118-158, 1983.
18. Petruzzello, S.J., Landers, D.M., Hatfield, B.D., et al. "A meta analysis on the anxiety reducing effects of acute and chronic exercise: Outcomes and mechanisms." *Sports Med* 11:143-182, 1991.
19. Reeves, D.L., Justesen, D.R., Levinson, D.M., et al. "Endogenous hyperthermia in normal human subjects: I. Experimental study of evoked potentials and reaction time." *Physiol Psychol* 13:258-267, 1985.
20. Rejeski, W.J. "Perceived exertion: An active or passive process?" *J Sport Psychol* 7:371-378, 1985.
21. Rejeski, W.J., Gregg, E., Thompson, A., et al. "The effects of varying doses of acute aerobic exercise on psychophysiological stress responses in highly trained cyclists." *J Sport Exerc Psychol* 13(2):188-199, 1991.
22. Rosenberg, M. *Conceiving the Self.* New York, NY: Basic, 1979.

23. Roskies, E., Seraganian, P., Oseasohn, R., et al. "The Montreal type A intervention project: Major findings." *Health Psychol* 5:45-69, 1986.

24. Salazar, W., Landers, D.M., Petruzzello, S.J., et al. "Effects of exercise on intellectual function: A meta analysis." Paper presented at the North American Society for the Psychology of Sport and Physical Activity. Monterey, CA, June 1991.

25. Schwartz, G.E., Weinberger, D.A., Singer, J.A. "Cardiovascular differentiation of happiness, sadness, anger, and fear following imagery and exercise." *Psychosom Med* 43:343-364, 1981.

26. Solomon, R.L., Corbit, J.D. "An opponent-process theory of motivation: II. Cigarette addiction." *J Abnormal Psychol* 81(2):158-171, 1973.

27. Sonstroem, R.J., Morgan, W.P. "Exercise and self-esteem: Rationale and model." *Med Sci Sports Exerc* 21:329-337, 1989.

28. Tomporowski, P.D., Ellis, N.R. "Effects of exercise on cognitive processes: A review." *Am Psychol* 99:338-346, 1986.

29. Williams, T.J., Krahenbuhl, G.S., Morgan, D.W. "Mood state and running economy in moderately trained male runners." Med Sci Sports *Exerc* 23:727-731, 1991.

30. Ziegler, S.G., Klinzing, J., Williamson, K. "The effects of two stress management training programs on cardiorespiratory efficiency." *J Sport Psychol* 4:280-289, 1982.

CHAPTER 7

••••••••••••••••••••••••••••••••

UNDERSTANDING CLOSED CHAIN EXERCISE*

by

Gary Gray, P.T.
• • •

> "The magic is not in the medicine, but in the patient's body—in the vis medicatrix natural, the recuperative or self-corrective energy of nature. What the treatment does is to stimulate natural functions or to remove what hinders them."
>
> C. S. Lewis
> from *Miracles*

*T*he aforementioned words of the late, renowned theologian and philosopher, C. S. Lewis, offer partial insight into a fundamental change which has begun to occur recently in the way medical professionals view the type of exercise necessary for effective rehabilitation of orthopaedic conditions. Traditionally, exercise has been perceived in a very structured way by the medical community. This perception involves introducing exercise into the rehab process on a restricted basis after a suitable (extended) period of time. Stabilize one part of the body (primarily while in a non-weight bearing position), and then exercise another part. This is an approach which has often been characterized by its proponents with such phrases as . . . "conservative" . . . the "proven" alternative . . . the "right" thing to do.

Regrettably, while the traditional approach to orthopaedic rehabilitation certainly appears to have been compatible with the comfort zone of those who relied on it, a growing body of both research and empirical evidence supports the conclusion that it is neither the "right thing to do" nor the "proven alternative." The traditional approach does not, in the words of C. S. Lewis, "stimulate natural functions." Rather, it requires the body to exercise in a very unnatural, non-functional manner.

---

* Note: Some of the material contained in this chapter is adapted from "Plane Sense," an article which appeared in *Fitness Management* 8(5):30-33, 1992.

Not only does non-functional exercise limit the degree of success which can be attained in the healing process, in many instances, it may even be counterproductive (injurious) to the entire rehab effort. Considerable evidence suggests that all other factors being equal, the more functional the exercise, the more effective the healing process.

CLOSED CHAIN VS. OPEN CHAIN EXERCISE

A strong argument can be made that the most practical way of evaluating the rehab effectiveness of exercise is to examine the relative position of the body during the exercise. Your body can be viewed as a chain. Your limbs (legs and arms) serve as the opposite ends of the chain. If either set of limbs is involved in supporting your weight (e.g., a squatting exercise in which your legs are bearing the weight of your body; a push-up in which your arms are partially shouldering the weight of your body), the physical endeavor is referred to as an example of a "closed chain exercise." The end segment of the chain is closed (e.g., fixed).

If the end segment of the chain (your body) is not fixed (e.g., free—not supporting the weight of your body), the exercise is termed an "open chain exercise." For numerous reasons, closed chain exercises are much more functional and effective in facilitating the healing process than open chain exercises.

The Greek philosopher Aristotle once (indirectly) provided a potential basis for comprehending the nature of closed chain exercise by stating, "The animal that moves makes its change of position by pressing that which is beneath it." This simple statement contains two elements which should be considered: the interaction between an animal (man) and its environment; and the way in which an animal organizes the pressing.

Closed chain exercise provides a natural way of exercising which involves functional movements. Functional movement is important because directly and indirectly it requires your body (joints, muscles, neurological system) to "conduct" itself as it does normally. As you exercise, your joints, muscles, and neurological system are required to react to each other as they do in real life. Muscles vary the degree to which they support and oppose each other depending on which (axial) cardinal plane(s) they happen to be in at any specific moment in time. In functional movement, joints incur different natural stresses, depending on the plane of movement, the velocity of the movement, and the type of loading to which they are exposed. Of equal importance, functional movement facilitates normal proprioceptive feedback. Your neurological system interacts with your musculoskeletal system in a coordinated fashion that produces safe and natural movement patterns.

One of the intrinsically important rules of rehabilitation is to create an environment for optimal healing. Closed chain exercise provides the means for individuals to safely engage in constructive rehab activities within a healing environment that focuses on the way bodies actually work.

Open chain exercises, on the other hand, involve isolated movements which impose artificial stresses (e.g., non-natural) on the body. The body is simply incapable of responding to such stresses in a functional way. As a result, the healing process is severely impeded—if not stopped.

Table 7-1 presents a comparative overview between open and closed chain rehabilitation techniques on twelve critical factors. A review of the differences between the two techniques strongly suggests that the substantial growth in the use of closed chain exercises in orthopaedic rehabilitation programs is well justified. Such a review also suggests that when individuals seek advice on how to rehab an injury, they should be encouraged to engage in closed chain exercises, as opposed to open chain.

Table 7-1. A Comparison Between Open and Closed Chain Rehabilitation Techniques for the Knee.

	Open Chain Exercise	Closed Chain Exercise
End Segment	Free	Fixed
Axis of Motion	Distal to the joint	Both proximal and distal to the joint
Muscle Contraction	Primarily concentric	Concentric, eccentric, and isometric
Movement	Isolated	Functional
Load	Artificial and sometimes abnormal	Normal physiological load through the skeletal system
Velocity	Sometimes predetermined; unsafe at upper limits	Variable according to exercise requirements
Stress/Strain	Biomechanically inconsistent within soft tissues	Biomechanically consistent within the soft tissues
Stabilization	Afforded through artificial means	Synergistic muscle contractions
Planes	Occurs in only one of the three cardinal planes	Occurs in all three cardinal planes, consistent with the motion of the joint & structures
Proprioception	Facilitates probable foreign and erroneous proprioceptive feedback	Facilitates normal proprioceptive feedback mechanisms
Rehabilitation Techniques	Limited to the design of the equipment being used	Unlimited potential
Rehabilitation Reaction	Non-integrated open and many times isolated event	Integrated chain reaction

The Value Of Closed Chain Exercise

The inherent value of closed chain exercise can be more clearly understood when the logic of noted endocrinologist Hans Selye's theory of stress adaptation is applied to the question of what type of exercises will have the most positive effect on the healing process. Selye found that the human body will gradually adapt to the stresses imposed upon it. If an individual imposes an artificial stress, the body adapts to that stress. Subsequently, when the body resumes functioning in a normal manner, the artificially-induced adaptation will be of minimal (if any) value. In all likelihood, if pain was present before the bout of open chain exercises, the pain will still exist if the body has otherwise failed to heal itself naturally over a specific period of time.

The validity of Selye's conclusions is even more apparent when the process of knee rehabilitation is considered. The knee is one area of the body which is commonly injured during participation in fitness and sport activities. Many fitness professionals erroneously advise any individual with knee pain to do leg extension exercises. In the first place, the cause of the individual's pain may originate in some other part of the body and have nothing to do with the muscles adjacent to the knee. Even if the pain was associated with some deficiency involving the muscles and attendant tissues and structures of the knee, having the individual perform an isolated exercise through a single plane of motion would make little, or no, sense. Rather, in the latter scenario, the individual should be counselled to perform controlled weight-bearing exercises (e.g., unweighted step-ups, partial squats, exercise on an independent step-action, mechanical stair climbing machine, etc.).

The value of performing controlled weight-bearing exercises is based on the concept that physiologically and biomechanically the human body is an extraordinarily complex entity in which the different parts interact according to the stresses imposed upon them in whatever position a particular structure is in at a given time. These positions vary from body area to body area, from moment to moment within any physical movement.

Biomechanists use the three basic cardinal planes (refer to Figure 7-1) of the body (frontal, sagittal, and transverse) as reference points. Unlike open chain exercise which isolates a part of the body during exercise to a single plane, closed chain exercise takes advantage of the fact that the human body is constantly in a triplane mode. At any given moment, forces (stresses) are being imposed on the body while it is in all three planes. Any effort to rehabilitate the body which is not based on this reality can be counterproductive to the healing process.

A Clear Choice

For reasons probably best appreciated by manufacturers of testing equipment which assess selected physiological and performance variables while individuals are performing open chain exercise, the question of which type of exercise—open chain vs. closed chain—is most appropriate for the rehabilitation process has traditionally been couched as an issue involving the conservative approach versus the aggressive approach. Aggressive has been unfairly perceived as taking undue risks, while the conservative approach has been viewed as the safe alternative. Neither categorization is justifiable. A more equitable way of looking at the entire matter is to examine the merits of a non-functional approach versus a functional approach. Artificial vs. natural. Make-do vs. can-do. Careful examination of the issue of open versus closed chain exercise would leave little doubt regarding which is the more functional method of rehabilitation. Closed chain exercise clearly makes good sense, as well as "plane sense." ❏

Figure 7-1. Schematic representation of the primary cardinal reference planes.

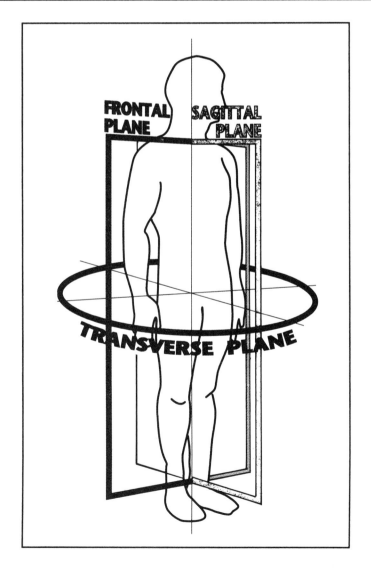

BIBLIOGRAPHY •

1. American Academy of Orthopaedic Surgeons. Symposium on the Athletic Knee: Surgical Repair and Reconstruction. St. Louis, MO: The C. V. Mosby Company, 1980.
2. Cailliet, R. Knee Pain and Disability. Philadelphia, PA: F. A. Davis Company, 1973.
3. Davies, G.J. et al. "Mechanisms of Selected Knee Injuries," *Phys Ther* 60:1590-1595, 1980.
4. Enoka, R.M. Neuromechanical Basis of Kinesiology. Champaign, IL: Human Kinetics Publishers, 1988.
5. Evans, F.G. (Ed). *Studies in the Anatomy and Function of Bones and Joints.* New York, NY: Wiley-Interscience, 1979.
6. Feagin, J.E. (Ed). *The Crucial Ligaments.* New York, NY: Churchill Livingstone, Inc., 1988.
7. Gray, G. *Chain Reaction.* (Unpublished Manual). Adrian, MI: Wynn Marketing, 1992.
8. Grieve, G. *Common Vertebrae Joint Problems.* New York, NY: Churchill Livingstone Inc., 1981.
9. MacConaill, M.A., Basmajian, J.V. *Muscles and Movements: A Basis for Human Kinesiology.* Baltimore, MD: Williams and Wilkins, 1969.
10. Maigne, R. *Orthopedic Medicine.* Springfield, IL: Charles C. Thomas, Publisher, 1976.
11. Mangine, R.E. (Ed). Physical *Therapy of the Knee.* New York, NY: Churchill Livingstone, 1988.
12. Mercier, L.R., Pettid, F.J. *Practical Orthopedics.* Chicago, IL: Year Book Medical Publishers, Inc., 1980.
13. Nordin, M., Frankel, V.H. Basic *Biomechanics of the Musculoskeletal System.* Philadelphia, PA: Lea and Febiger, 1989.
14. Rasch, P.J. *Kinesiology and Applied Anatomy.* Philadelphia, PA: Lea and Febiger, 1989.
15. Zuidema, G.D. (Ed). *The Johns Hopkins Atlas of Human Functional Anatomy*, 2nd Ed. Baltimore, MD: The Johns Hopkins University Press, 1980.

CHAPTER 8

• •

UNDERSTANDING GRADED EXERCISE TESTING

by

George J. Holland, Ph.D.
and
Steven F. Loy, Ph.D.

• • •

*O*nce you reach a decision to start exercising, your physician may recommend that you undergo a graded exercise test (GXT) before you begin your exercise regimen, a procedure which is commonly referred to as an exercise stress test. Such a recommendation from your physician may raise a number of questions in your mind regarding a GXT: What does a GXT involve? Why should you undergo a GXT? Is it safe? What information does it provide? Etc. This chapter addresses the aforementioned questions and other relevant issues concerning graded exercise testing in an attempt to remove much of the confusion and mystery that sometimes surrounds this increasingly utilized evaluative procedure.*

WHAT A GXT INVOLVES

A GXT can be administered in a variety of locations, including a physician's office, at a hospital, or at a professionally supervised health and fitness facility. Regardless of where a GXT is administered, special equipment to handle any medical emergency that may arise and a sufficient number of appropriately trained professionals must be present. According to the guidelines established by the American Heart Association (AHA), all individuals who administer GXTs should be trained in cardiopulmonary resuscitation (CPR—see Appendix B), and at least one of the technicians in the testing area should also be trained and certified in advanced cardiac life support. Also, in accordance with AHA guidelines, a physician should be on the premises (e.g., in the building) at all times.

---

* Individuals interested in obtaining information concerning the administration of a GXT should refer to the bibliography for this chapter.

To prepare for a GXT, you should abstain from food, tobacco, alcohol and caffeine for a minimum of three hours before your test—since all of these substances affect your physiological responses to exercise. In addition, you should wear comfortable shoes (e.g., sneakers, walking shoes, etc.) and loose-fitting clothes (e.g., a t-shirt and gym shorts). If you are a woman, it is advisable that you wear a loose-fitting blouse that (preferably) buttons down the front—this permits easier attachment of the ECG electrodes. Women, undergoing a GXT, should not wear nylon bras (since nylon material tends to interfere with the ECG tracings).

Prior to the start of a GXT, a resting electrocardiogram (ECG) is performed to check for cardiac abnormalities that exist in the absence of "stress" and to provide a basis for comparison with your physiological responses during the exercise session. Both resting blood pressure and heart rate are assessed and monitored throughout a GXT. Electrodes (sensors) are placed on your chest during a resting ECG. These sensors remain in place during a GXT, so that the rhythm and electrical activity of your heart can be monitored continuously throughout the GXT. At rest, an ECG may indicate that your heart is receiving adequate amounts of blood and oxygen, but when you're stressed (i.e., during exercise), an ECG may reveal signs that your heart is receiving insufficient amounts of blood and oxygen.

A variety of modalities (e.g., a treadmill, a stationary cycle, a stair climbing machine, etc.) can be used to provide the exercise stress. The motor-driven treadmill is the device most commonly used in the United States for graded exercise testing. In general, a GXT initially involves placing a relatively low level of exercise-induced stress on your cardiovascular system. Subsequent increases in work demand are then gradually incorporated into the exercise protocol that you are required to perform by raising either the speed or grade (incline) of the treadmill. Because the goal of a GXT is simply to determine the capability limits of your cardiovascular system, you need not worry about the treadmill reaching "warp" speed or being raised to a grade that simulates Mount Everest.

Two different types of GXTs can be administered. One is referred to as a symptom-limited maximal GXT and the other as a submaximal GXT. The symptom-limited maximal GXT is the more common of the two types of GXTs and involves the progressive increase of the exercise intensity until you display signs or symptoms of exertional intolerance. The submaximal GXT, on the other hand, progressively increases the level of exercise intensity until you reach some predetermined end point (e.g., 85% of your maximum heart rate) or until a sign or symptom of exertional intolerance occurs before the end point has been reached.

WHO SHOULD HAVE A STRESS TEST?

The current guidelines of AHA indicate that if you are under age 40 (male and female) and undergo a normal physical examination, which indicates no symptoms of cardiovascular disease, no major coronary risk factors, no physical findings (including murmurs and hypertension), you can be considered free of disease and do not require GXT before undertaking a new exercise regimen. If you are 40 years of age or older, have had an abnormal physical examination (murmurs, etc.) or possess two or more coronary risk factors, you should have a GXT before embarking on a vigorous exercise program (refer to Table 2-1 for a listing of the major coronary risk factors).

In guidelines recently revised by the American College of Sports Medicine (ACSM), a GXT is not recommended prior to initiation of an exercise program if you are an asymptomatic male 40 years or younger, or female 50 years or younger. If you are an older asymptomatic adult (males 40 plus, females 50 plus), you may initiate a moderate exercise regimen (intensity 40-60% VO_2 max) without a GXT. A GXT is recommended for all older adults planning a vigorous exercise program (intensity greater than 60% VO_2 max).

The ACSM uses the same criteria of two or more major coronary risk factors as the basis for recommending a GXT prior to an individual's beginning an exercise program. Gradual moderate exercise is, however, permitted without a GXT for individuals without coronary artery disease (CAD) symptoms, but with two or more CAD risk factors. Individuals with two or more risk factors, but without symptoms, should undergo a GXT before vigorous exercise. The ACSM recommendations regarding who should be required to take a GXT and the attendant level of requisite supervision are outlined in chapter 2 (refer to Table 2-3).

How Safe Is A GXT?

Like most medical procedures, a GXT is not without some risk. The risk can be minimized by proper screening and by having the test administered by properly trained personnel. As stated previously, personnel involved in conducting a GXT should be thoroughly familiar with the equipment and trained to handle emergency situations should they arise. Although untoward events (e.g., heart attacks) are well publicized, they are extremely rare (less than one per every 500 symptom-limited GXTs). The risk of a fatal clinical complication is much lower (less than 1 in 10,000).

What Information Does A GXT Provide?

In the early stages of CAD, individuals usually do not exhibit symptoms of coronary insufficiency while either at rest or during nonstrenuous activity. During exercise, however, signs or symptoms of CAD often become manifest, as the demands for oxygen increase beyond what the diseased arteries can supply. If the oxygen demand and supply imbalance is relatively large, it can cause anginal chest pain—a hallmark sign of CAD. Smaller oxygen imbalances can cause changes in heart rate, blood pressure, and heart rhythm and may elicit changes on the ECG. An abnormal ECG during a GXT is only suggestive that a cardiac problem is present since the results of such tests are not always accurate. Approximately 16% of GXTs result in false positives (i.e., the test erroneously indicates that an individual has heart disease). Unfortunately, a higher proportion (34%) of false negative (i.e., the test incorrectly indicates that an individual is free of heart disease) GXT results occur. Accordingly, when evaluating your test results, your physician will consider all of the following: how long and through what stage you exercised, what your heart rate and blood pressure responses were, whether any rhythm disturbances of heart occurred and when they occurred, whether any ECG abnormalities appeared, and how you looked and felt.

AFTER THE GXT

Once you have taken a GXT, you should discuss the results with your doctor. If no problems are discovered, the information obtained from the GXT should be used to help design an appropriate exercise program for your specific goals, needs, interests, and fitness level. Should your physician feel that your stress test was not accurate, or was inconclusive, he or she may recommend a thallium exercise stress test* in order to improve diagnostic accuracy.

Remember, it is impossible to "flunk" a GXT. If a problem is detected, it is much better to identify it in the controlled setting of your physician's office, a hospital, an exercise science laboratory, or a medically supervised health and fitness club than in your own home. Finally, no matter who you are, you can benefit from participating in an exercise program based on the information obtained from a properly conducted GXT. ❑

---

* A radioactive dye (thallium-201) is injected into your arm and its passage is traced through your heart during a graded exercise test to more definitively determine if CAD is present, and if so, to what degree of severity. For more information on thallium exercise stress testing refer to items 3, 6, 13, and 15 in the bibliography.

BIBLIOGRAPHY •••

1. American College of Cardiology/American Heart Association. "Guidelines for exercise testing." *Am J Cardiol* 8:725-738, 1986.
2. American College of Sports Medicine. *Guidelines for Graded Exercise Testing and Prescription,* 4th Ed. Philadelphia, PA: Lea & Febiger, 1991.
3. American College of Sports Medicine. *Resource Manual for Graded Exercise Testing and Prescription.* Philadelphia, PA: Lea & Febiger, 1988.
4. American Heart Association. "Exercise Standards." *Circulation* 82:2286-2322, 1990.
5. Ellestad, M.H. *Stress testing: Principles and practice,* 3rd Ed. Philadelphia, PA: F. A. Davis Company, 1986.
6. Foster, C. "Stress testing: Directions for the future." *Sports Med* 6:11-22, 1988.
7. Franklin, B.A., Gordon, S., Timmis, G.C. (Eds). *Exercise in modern medicine.* Baltimore, MD: Williams & Wilkins, 1989.
8. Froelicher, V.F. *Exercise and the Heart: Clinical Concepts.* Chicago, IL: Year Book Publishers, 1987.
9. Froelicher, V.F. *Exercise testing and training.* Chicago, IL: Year Book Publishers, Inc., 1983.
10. Gibbons, L., Blair, S.N., Kohl, H.W., et al. "The Safety of Maximal Exercise Testing." *Circulation* 80:846-854, 1989.
11. Holland, G.J., Heng, M.K., Weber, F. "Exercise Testing for Asymptomatic Adults." *Cardiovasc Rev Reports* 9(6):38-40, 1988.
12. Holland, G.J., Hoffman, J.J., Vincent, W., et al. "Treadmill vs. Steptreadmill Ergometry." *Phys Sportsmed* 18:79-85, 1990.
13. Holland, G.J., Weber, F., Weng, M.K., et al. "Maximal steptreadmill exercise and treadmill exercise by patients with coronary heart disease: A comparison." *J Cardiopulmonary Rehabil* 8:58-68, 1988.
14. Iskandrian, A.S., Wasserman, L.A., Anderson, G.S., et al. "Merits of stress thallium-201 myocardial perfusion imaging in patients with inconclusive exercise electrocardiograms: Correlation with coronary arteriograms." *Am J Cardiol* 46:553-558, 1980.
15. Pollock, M.L., Wilmore, J.H. *Exercise in Health and Disease; Evaluation and Prescription for Prevention and Rehabilitation,* 2nd Ed. Philadelphia, PA: W. B. Saunders Company, 1990.
16. Ritchie, J.L., Trobaugh, G.B., Hamilton, G.W., et al. "Myocardial imaging with thallium-201 at rest and during exercise: Comparison with coronary arteriography and resting and stress electrocardiography." *Circulation* 56:66-71, 1977.
17. Skinner, J.S. (Ed). *Exercise Testing and Exercise Prescription for Special Cases.* Philadelphia, PA: Lea & Febiger, 1987.

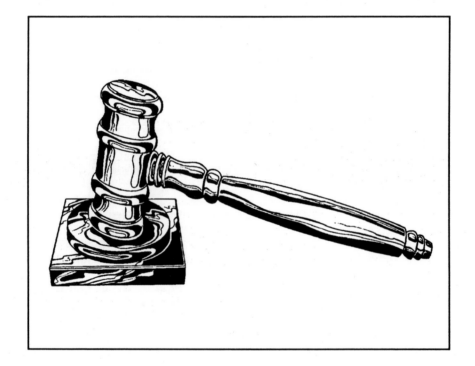

CHAPTER 9

• •

LEGAL CONSIDERATIONS IN GRADED EXERCISE TESTING AND EXERCISE PRESCRIPTION*

by
David L. Herbert, J.D.
and
William G. Herbert, Ph.D.

• • •

*A*s was discussed in chapter 8, graded exercise (stress) testing (GXTs) procedures are assessment techniques which are widely used for a variety of purposes. In general, the two main uses of GXTs involve exercise testing and exercise prescription. Medical professionals, for example, have traditionally employed GXTs to diagnose the status of individuals with known or suspected coronary heart disease. In fact, the use of exercise stress testing procedures within the medical provider section has grown dramatically in the past few years. The rise in the popularity of GXTs within the medical community is reinforced by recent statistics which indicate that GXTs are currently used by medical personnel as a prognostic indicator for almost half of all acute heart patients.[1]

The use of GXTs to provide much of the basis for exercise prescription has also grown in popularity in recent years. Prescribing exercise based on a thorough analysis of baseline GXT results is frequently employed for relatively healthy individuals with a primary interest in fitness, as well as for individuals with a medically related condition.

The sharp increase in the use of GXTs has also given rise to a number of rather significant legal issues associated with such evaluative practices. These issues

---

*Note: This chapter is focused specifically for those professionals involved in conducting graded exercise testing or prescribing exercise. Individuals with a general interest in fitness, however, may find this information enlightening.

[1] " *TRENDS*, "Dramatic Increase in Diagnostic Testing for MI Patients Reported," *THE EXERCISE STANDARDS & MALPRACTICE REPORTED* 2(2):28, 1988.

center upon: (1) the relative safety of stress testing procedures; (2) the propriety of non-physician personnel carrying out such procedures; and (3) the legal risks associated with the performance of these tests.

SAFETY CONCERNS ASSOCIATED WITH TESTING

In 1971, the results of a large-scale study of exercise stress testing procedures were reported by P. Rochmis and H. Blackburn.[2] An analysis of the results of this study, as well as other studies that have been conducted since, indicate a rather low incidence of serious risk associated with GXT procedures (approximately one-half to one in 10,000 tests).

Most individuals within the medical community consider GXTs to be relatively safe, especially when supervised by a physician. Many individuals also believe that these tests may be carried out by appropriately trained/certified non-physicians.[3] Some professionals, however, feel that GXTs should only be conducted or supervised under the direction of a physician.[4] The preliminary results of a recently completed analysis of a twelve-year study of more than 41,000 GXTs indicates that specifically trained non-physicians may safely perform GXTs, at least in a hospital setting.[5]

Prescribing exercise on the basis of GXT results can involve a myriad of safety concerns. Each of the concerns is inextricably related in many instances to how well the GXT is administered and how accurately the GXT results are interpreted. Improper exercise prescription or exercise prescription without the development of adequate baseline information can result in participant injury and even death. Unfortunately, the diverse settings within which exercise prescriptions are developed are not (as a rule) offered the opportunity for uniform statistics to be compiled regarding the safety of specific prescriptions for particular patient populations. Medico-legal fact patterns have arisen, however, which should provide an appropriate basis for examining and better understanding the GXT safety issues involving exercise prescription, as well as testing procedures.

---

[2] "Exercise Tests: A Survey of Procedures, Safety and Litigation Experience in Approximately 170,000 Tests," *JAMA*, 217:1061-1066, 1971.

[3] *BLESSEY*, "Exercise Testing By Non-Physician Health Care Professionals: Complication Rates, Clinical Competencies and Future Trends," *THE EXERCISE STANDARDS AND MALPRACTICE REPORTER.*

[4] *GIBBONS M.D.*, "Editorial - The Safety of Maximal Exercise Testing," *J. CARDIOPULMONARY REHABIL*, 7:277, 1987.

[5] *NEWS & REPORTS*, "New Study: Specially Trained Non-Physicians Can Safely Supervise GXTs," *THE EXERCISE STANDARDS AND MALPRACTICE REPORTER* 5(1):10, 1991.

THE PRACTICE AND UNAUTHORIZED PRACTICE OF MEDICINE

The practice of medicine is universally regulated by state licensing laws defining the practice, specifying who may conduct the activities and under what circumstances.[6] Those individuals who engage in such activities without proper licensure run the risk of being charged with the crime of the unauthorized practice of medicine (generally a misdemeanor), as well as having their conduct, in the event of some untoward event and suit, judged in accordance with the standard of care for those practicing medicine, Id. Non-physicians cannot escape such a comparison without having liability attached to their conduct.

In the exercise field, many potential concerns arise that are related to the unauthorized practice of medicine. This situation is particularly true for testing procedures and exercise prescriptions. Generally, if GXTs are carried out within a medical setting and for medically related purposes, or if a prescription of exercise is provided for the treatment of a disease, condition, or infirmity, then nearly universal agreement exists that those carrying out such procedures are engaged in the practice of medicine. In the event that such procedures are carried out for non-medical purposes in a non-health care setting (e.g., for fitness assessment evaluations and/or by non-medical personnel), then in all likelihood, such procedures are not medical in nature. It is in those areas, between these two extremes, that questions and potential legal concerns arise. These concerns are complicated by the diversity of state laws and administrative regulations impacting the practice of medicine and other allied health care professions.

The State of North Carolina Medical Examiners, for example, issued a statement in June 1987 declaring: "When a non-physician administers a graded exercise test, the standard of care in North Carolina is that a physician is to be in the room or the immediate area.[7]" Obviously, expressions of concern similar to this one can raise significant legal issues as to who can properly conduct GXTs, and under what circumstances.

Little doubt exists that the debate regarding the propriety of a non-physician performing GXTs and/or prescribing physical activity is certain to continue for the foreseeable future. Concurrently, it is also reasonably certain that this debate will continue to be impacted by a variety of statements from a myriad of prominent professional associations. These statements concerning the applicable standards of practice will impact the provision of service and may affect court interpretation of state legislative practice statutes and regulations. The interrelationship of these laws and professional practice standards are brought into sharp focus in various court proceedings dealing with issues related to informed consent, negligence and malpractice. A comprehensive examination of these issues points out the potential

---

[6] *HERBERT & HERBERT, LEGAL ASPECTS OF PREVENTIVE AND REHABILITATIVE EXERCISE PROGRAMS*, 2nd Ed., 113-144 (Professional Reports Corporation, Canton, Ohio, 1989).

[7] *TRENDS*, "Physician Must be Present For Administration of Graded Exercise Tests," *THE EXERCISE STANDARDS & MALPRACTICE REPORTER*, 1(5):75, 1987.

legal factors that should be considered either when administering GXTs or when prescribing exercise.

INFORMED CONSENT

The law of informed consent requires—among other things—that every patient be informed of the material and relevant risks associated with any contemplated medical procedure, before the procedure is commenced. In quasi-medical or non-medical settings, the medical doctrine of informed consent may or may not apply. Some form of consent, however, will always be required for any procedure involving human clients.

In both the settings involving either the testing of exercise subjects or the provision of exercise prescriptions, the law has impacted the informed consent process. For example, in the 1985 case of Hedgecorth v. United States,[8] an elderly patient underwent a physician-supervised GXT at a VA hospital. He had a significant adverse medical history and had recently undergone another GXT procedure at another facility, the results of which were not obtained by the VA hospital. While he underwent a pre-test informed consent process, no disclosures as to either risk of stroke or blindness due to stroke were disclosed to him by his physicians. During the test, he suffered a stroke and later blindness due to the stroke. He and his wife subsequently brought suit contending that the physicians were negligent in their provision of information to him and that the consent process was thus void, rendering the physicians liable for all adverse consequences which occurred related to the procedure. A jury returned a verdict of nearly one million dollars to the patient and his wife. While the risk of stroke and the resultant risk of blindness due to stroke associated with GXT procedures must be considered minute, the case has resulted in a "rethinking" of the informed consent process for such procedures. In fact, it may have provided the impetus for the recent decision of the American College of Sports Medicine (ACSM) to revise its recommended informed consent disclosure form to include the risk of stroke.[9]

In another GXT-related informed consent case, a plaintiff's estate brought suit contending that the physician did not disclose the risk of death to the decedent and, as a consequence, the consent was void, rendering the physician liable for the untoward event which occurred after the test.[10] Despite these contentions, a jury returned a defense verdict upon the estate's lawsuit. A subsequent appeal

---

[8] Hedgecorth v. United States, 618 F. Suppl. 627 (E. D. Mo. 1985), analyzed in HERBERT, "Informed Consent Documents For Stress Testing To Comport With Hedgecorth vs. United States," THE EXERCISE STANDARDS AND MALPRACTICE REPORTER 1(6):81-88, 1987.

[9] HERBERT, "Sample Informed Consent Forms From the AHA, AACVPR and the ACSM," THE EXERCISE STANDARDS AND MALPRACTICE REPORTER 5(1):7-8, 1991.

[10] Smogor vs. Enke, 874 F. 2d 295 (5th Cir. 1989), analyzed in HERBERT, "Exercise Stress Testing Lawsuit Results in Defense Verdict," THE EXERCISE STANDARDS AND MALPRACTICE REPORTER 4(2):23-24, 1990.

resulted in a finding that a written informed consent form had been signed by the decedent which specifically "informed him of the risk of death."[11] Consequently, the defense verdict was upheld. Quite a different result could have occurred had no such statement been contained within the informed consent document. Sample informed consent forms for GXT procedures which do not utilize full disclosures including the risk of stroke and death in addition to other more traditional risks, should be viewed with cautious circumspection.[12]

The informed consent doctrine also impacts the prescription process. Risks associated with prescribed activities should be reviewed and discussed with patients prior to providing advice as to particular exercise. Shortcomings in this area can lead to significant litigation. For example, in the Utah case of Mikkelsen v. Haslam,[13] the plaintiff, who was affected with a congenitally dislocated right hip, sought physician advice and recommendation as to her condition. She subsequently underwent a total hip replacement and a period of rehabilitation. She contended that her physician eventually endorsed her participation in snow skiing. Later, during her participation in the activity, she fractured her femur and fell. Evidence indicated that the injury was due to a deteriorating condition of the bone. She subsequently brought suit contending that the physician was negligent in his provision of advice. The issues raised in the case will ultimately be decided by a jury trial.[14]

In another case, Contino v. Lucille Roberts Health Spa,[15] a chiropractor prescribed aerobic dance exercise for a back patient. She subsequently sought spa membership to engage in the recommended activity. She fell while doing the activity and later brought suit against the facility contending she was injured due to overcrowding, improper supervision and negligent leadership. The facility joined the chiropractor who prescribed the activity in the litigation. In considering the chiropractor's potential liability, the court determined that the pleadings in the case set forth an "ample basis" for prescriber liability based upon the allegation that the chiropractor's advice was negligent.[16]

A number of other cases involving GXT procedures and the prescription of exercise, but not entailing factors specifically related to informed consent, should

---

[11] Smoger vs. Enke, p. 297.

[12] HERBERT "Sample Informed Consent Forms From the AHA, AACVPR and the ACSM," supra.

[13] Mikkelsen v. Haslam, 764 p. 2d 1384, 1988.

[14] "Provider's Alleged Advice To Ski May Result In Liability," THE EXERCISE STANDARDS AND MALPRACTICE REPORTER 4(1):13-14, 1990.

[15] Contino v. Lucille Roberts Health Spa, 509 NYS 2d 369 (A.D. 2 Dept. 1986).

[16] LITIGATION AND COURT RULINGS, "Chiropractor's Advice To Patient To Take Aerobic Dance Class May Be Negligent," THE EXERCISE STANDARDS AND MALPRACTICE REPORTER 1(3):45-47, 1987.

also be considered. These cases, while not subject to common classification, deal with issues of negligence and malpractice.

NEGLIGENCE AND MALPRACTICE

Negligence is generally regarded as a failure to govern one's conduct to a generally accepted standard or duty. A cause of action upon the basis of negligence is established upon proof of DUTY, BREACH OF DUTY, PROXIMATELY CAUSING HARM/DAMAGE TO ANOTHER. Such a cause of action may be based upon a substandard act or an omission to act. Malpractice is simply negligence committed in the course and scope of a professional, patient/client relationship.

For GXT and exercise prescription procedures, a number of issues and cases dealing with negligence/malpractice have arisen. Examining these issues and cases can lead to a better understanding of the legal factors associated with same. In the "classic" exercise testing case of Tart vs. McGann,[17] the patient/plaintiff underwent a physician-supervised GXT procedure as part of his regular physical process to maintain his commercial airline pilot's license. During the fourth stage of the test, the plaintiff pilot testified that he began to feel tired and fatigued, but in light of the physician's encouragement, continued on with the test. After completing the test, he suffered a heart attack and brought suit contending that the physician should have terminated the test due to his outward but nonverbalized manifestations of fatigue.

Of particular importance during the jury trial was the question of the duty of the physician to stop the test in light of the pilot's facial expressions of fatigue. While expert testimony differed on physician's duty to terminate the test under such circumstances, the standards of the American Heart Association (AHA) were used to "judge" provider conduct in the case. Although a defense verdict was eventually rendered, the plaintiff received a substantial settlement. Thereafter, the provider population began to grapple with the issue of physician obligation to stop such procedures based upon evaluations of the patient's level of fatigue and distress.[18]

In other GXT-related cases, negligence/malpractice claims have been put forth dealing with a variety of issues, including improper placement of electrocardiographic leads, allegedly resulting in missed ST segment changes,[19] falls from

---

[17] Tart vs. McGann, 697 F. 2d 75 (2d Cir. 1982).

[18] EDELMAN, "The Case of Tart vs. McCann: Legal Implications Associated With Exercise Stress Testing," THE EXERCISE STANDARDS AND MALPRACTICE REPORTER 1(2):21-26, 1987.

[19] Kolodney v. U.S., U.S. Dist. Ct., Maryland, 1975, CIVIL CASE NO. M-74-108.

treadmills, or inappropriate supervision or instruction as to their use. [20],[21],[22]

One of the most significant cases of alleged negligence dealing with the prescription of physical activity involves a California malpractice arbitration case focusing upon the death of a patient, Ricardo Camerena. Mr. Camerena was a 40-year old patient who sought a physical examination and clearance prior to starting an exercise program. While he was given a physical, a resting electrocardiogram and blood tests, no GXT was performed. Following completion of this examination no restrictions were placed upon his activities. He died shortly thereafter while jogging, due to a heart attack.

His estate subsequently brought a claim against the physician contending that the physician was negligent in not conducting a GXT to screen him for silent ischemia prior to the decedent's commencement of activity. The arbitration panel ruled in favor of the estate and awarded the family $500,000.00. The plaintiff's lawyer subsequently claimed that the case stood for the proposition that **all** men 40 years of age or older required a GXT prior to beginning such activities. Some practitioners have contended that such testing is now a necessary defensive medicare tactic.[23] While such contentions have been strongly contested by some individual practitioners in the medical profession[24] and questioned by some subsequent statements of professional societies,[25] the substantial possibility always exists for such claims to be brought upon the prescription of activity which is not preceded and based upon the results and interpretation of a properly conducted and performed GXT.[26]

Negligence/malpractice cases are greatly affected by statements of professional associations. These statements, oftentimes referred to as standards, parameters of practice, or guidelines, can impact the provision of service, as well as the

---

[20] Figure World v. Farley, 680 S.W. 2d 33 (Tex. App. 3 Dist. 1986), analyzed in *LITIGATION AND COURT RULINGS*: "Participant Injuries Suffered While On Jogging Treadmill Can Be Facility's Responsibility," *THE EXERCISE STANDARDS AND MALPRACTICE REPORTER* 1(4) 161, 1987.

[21] Malkiewicz v. Overlia, No. 470493 (1987), *LITIGATION AND COURT RULINGS*, "Treadmill Fall Results In Defense Verdict," *THE EXERCISE STANDARDS AND MALPRACTICE REPORTER* 2(2):30, 1988.

[22] Tucker v. Trotter Treadmills, Inc., 779 P. 2d 524 (Mont. 1989), *LITIGATION AND COURT RULINGS*, "Suit Against Treadmill Manufacturer Dismissed," *THE EXERCISE STANDARDS AND MALPRACTICE REPORTER* 4(1):11-12, 1990.

[23] *KEIFETZ AND WATKINS*, "Routine Stress Tests Now Defensive Tactic," *MEDICAL TRENDS* 30(14):1, 8 (1989).

[24] *ASSEY*, "Screening for Silent Myocardial Ischemia," *AFB* 38(6):13-146, 1988.

[25] *AHA/ACC/ACP*, "Clinical Competence In Exercise Testing," *CIRCULATION* 82(5):1884-1888, 1990.

[26] *LITIGATION AND COURT RULES*: "Are GXTs Required For Screening Of All Men Over 40?," *THE EXERCISE STANDARDS AND MALPRACTICE REPORTER* 2(2):30, 1988.

outcome of negligence/malpractice suits. As a result, they must be considered within the scope of any review of this subject.

STANDARDS OF PRACTICE

The provision of services through GXT procedures or by way of exercise prescription is greatly affected by the written expression of the standard of care for these services. Standards of practice for these services have been developed and promulgated by the ACSM and the AHA, as well as the American Association for Cardiovascular and Pulmonary Rehabilitation (AACVPR), and the American College of Cardiology (ACC), as well as several other professional associations and groups—all of which impose written expressions as to the standard of care.[27],[28],[29],[30] While each set of standards may be written to one degree or another by reference to a particular perspective, each greatly impacts the delivery of service, as well as the standard of care, owed to various patient populations. New standards have been developed by almost all of these organizations as of early 1991. Professionals practicing in these areas must be familiar with these standards and the developing effect of these standards on the provision of related services.

CONCLUSION

Legal concerns abound for those delivering exercise testing or prescription services. A familiarization with the legal concerns associated with these procedures as well as the standards of practice which impact same, can only assist the practitioner in avoiding patient/participant injury and claim, in addition to helping preclude a conflict with the legal system. Providers must stay abreast of professional developments in relevant areas and become familiar with what is expected of them in the course of carrying out their duties and responsibilities toward their patient population. Anything less may result in patient injury or death, and concomitant claims and suits. ❏

---

[27] ACSM, *GUIDELINES FOR EXERCISE TESTING AND PRESCRIPTION*, 4TH ED. (Lea & Febiger, Philadelphia, PA, 1991).

[28] AHA: Fletcher, et al., "Exercise Standards: A Statement for Health Professionals From the American Heart Association," *CIRCULATION* 82(6):2286-2322, 1990.

[29] AACVPR: *GUIDELINES FOR CARDIAC REHABILITATION PROGRAMS* (Human Kinetics, Champaign, IL, 1991).

[30] ACC: "Recommendations of the American College of Cardiology on Cardiovascular Rehabilitation," *CARDIOLOGY* 15(2):4-5, March 1986.

CHAPTER 10

● ●

ASSESSING PHYSICAL FITNESS

by

Victor Ben-Ezra, Ph.D.

● ● ●

*A*ssessing your level of physical fitness is a process which can serve several important functions. First and foremost, it can provide you with a "status report" regarding your level of each of the major components of physical fitness. The results of your fitness evaluation can also be used to identify any particular deficiencies you might have. By identifying your (fitness) strengths and weaknesses, your training program can be modified to address specific shortcomings. Fitness tests can also help evaluate the progress you are making in your exercise program. If, for example, you are not experiencing an appreciable level of improvement in a particular component of fitness, you may need to adjust your exercise prescription. Finally, the results of fitness testing can be used to motivate you to continue exercising. Positive feedback emanating from the results of your exercise efforts can reinforce your attitudes towards the value of and the necessity for such efforts.

The steps involved in evaluating your level of physical fitness can vary in their degree of complexity. Fitness testing can be conducted in both laboratory and non-laboratory settings. Tests of physical fitness can also differ in how difficult they are to administer, how much equipment is involved, how expensive they are to perform and how many and what kind of personnel are required to administer them.

Whatever type of physical fitness test you select, it should meet certain criteria. It should accurately measure what it is supposed to measure (i.e., it must have *validity*). It should provide consistent results (i.e., it must exhibit repeatability—*reliability*). It should provide the foundation for a comparison (i.e., the test results must be able to be interpreted or evaluated on the basis of *norms*). Finally, it should be *user-friendly* (i.e., the test should be relatively easy to administer, time-efficient and provide easy-to-understand feedback to the individual taking it).

This chapter presents an overview of several of the basic methods for assessing each of the four primary components of physical fitness: body composition, aerobic fitness, muscular fitness (strength and endurance) and flexibility. The assessment techniques for each component are grouped into two categories: laboratory and non-laboratory tests. All factors considered, as a general rule, physical fitness testing in a laboratory yields more accurate measurements, involves more expense and difficulty in administering, and requires specifically trained personnel. Non-laboratory tests, on the other hand, are usually easy to administer and can be conducted in a wide variety of locations, although they provide results which are comparatively less accurate than tests performed in a laboratory setting.

BEFORE THE TEST

Before you take a physical fitness test, certain guidelines should be followed to ensure both your safety and the accuracy of the test results. You should wear comfortable, loose fitting clothing during the test. You should avoid food, tobacco, alcohol, and coffee for at least three hours prior to taking the test, and not exercise prior to the test on the day of the test. In addition, you should try to get a sufficient amount of sleep the night before. If the test involves having your blood analyzed, you should avoid consuming alcohol and exercising vigorously for a full day prior to the test and not eat for 12 hours before a test in which your blood is to be analyzed.

THE ORDER OF THE FITNESS TESTS

Depending on what fitness components are to be evaluated, the organization of the testing session is very important. If all components are to be assessed in a single session, body composition measures should be taken first, followed (in order) by aerobic fitness, muscular fitness and flexibility. For example, taking a graded exercise (stress) test (GXT) after assessing muscular fitness and flexibility (both of which elevate heart rate) can produce an inaccurate reading of the status of an individual's aerobic fitness level—particularly when submaximal tests are used. Body composition is usually assessed first because other forms of exercise testing can influence it. If the testing protocol involves assessing certain measures at rest (e.g., heart rate, blood pressure and blood analysis), such measures should be taken before the fitness testing begins.

BODY COMPOSITION*

Body composition is often defined as the ratio of fat to fat-free mass in your body. For the most part, fat-free mass is comprised of muscle, bone, water and

---

* Note: The author would like to thank Phil Buckenmeyer for his contributions to the sections on body composition and flexibility.

protein, while adipose tissue makes up the fat mass component of your body. Determining whether you have a ratio appropriate for good health is important since excessive fat (obesity) has been shown to be a risk factor for certain diseases, such as coronary heart disease, hypertension and diabetes. Assessing body composition can be accomplished through a variety of laboratory and non-laboratory methods.

LABORATORY TESTS FOR BODY COMPOSITION

The most widely used procedure in a laboratory setting for assessing body composition is hydrostatic weighing—commonly referred to as *underwater weighing*. Underwater weighing involves determining whole body density by measuring how much you weigh when you are totally submerged in water. Your weight underwater and on land are then used in an equation which has been developed to predict body density. Such a calculation is possible because fat and lean tissue do not have the same level of density. Fat tissue is less dense. As a result, an individual with a high percentage of fat weighs less underwater than an individual with the same weight on land but with a lower percentage of body fat. Despite its accuracy, hydrostatic weighing is not widely used because the technique is relatively inefficient time-wise, involves relatively expensive equipment, and requires trained, experienced technicians to administer.

Other laboratory-based techniques for assessing body composition include: potassium-K counting, measuring total body electrical conductivity (TOBEC), measuring the excretion muscle metabolites (creatinine and 3-methyl histidine), measuring total body water, ultrasound, computed tomography, dual photon absorptiometry, bioelectrical impedance, and infrared interactance.[*] While each of these techniques has a few desirable features and exhibits some degree of promise as an assessment tool, none has been found to be sufficiently practical to warrant its widespread use.

NON-LABORATORY TESTS FOR BODY COMPOSITION

The most widely used method for assessing body composition is based on the thickness of skinfolds. Skinfold testing involves using a calibrated tool (commonly referred to as skinfold calipers) to measure how thick the fat folds are on selected body segments.

The usual procedure for measuring skinfolds involves simply grasping the skin and its underlying fat with the thumb and index finger into a double fold. With the other hand, the arms of the caliper are opened and gently closed over the skinfold which is being held by the opposite hand. The tips of the caliper arms are

---

[*] Editors' Note: Bioelectrical impedance and infrared interactance are becoming more widely used in non-laboratory settings. The validity and reliability of these two techniques for analyzing body composition, however, remain the subject of scientific debate.

placed approximately one-half inch from the thumb and index finger. The caliper then grasps the skinfold for about 2-3 seconds. A value representing the relative "thickness" of the measured skinfold is then noted and recorded in millimeters. The caliper tips are subsequently released from the skinfold, and the person doing the testing lets go of the skinfold. Three to four trial measurements at each site are recommended. The average of the measurements is then used.

Several equations have been developed over the years that employ a variety of skinfold sites to estimate body density and predict percent body fat. These equations are gender and age specific and are designed to be used only with a similar population from which they were derived. Of equal importance, each equation is based on specific sites and requires that specified techniques for measuring the skinfolds at each site be employed.

The following are examples of equations that have been successfully employed over the years for men ages 18-61 years and women ages 18-55 years (using Lange calipers) to assess body composition:

Men
- Body density = $1.1093800 - 0.0008267(x1) = 0.0000016(x1)2 - 0.0002574(x2)$.
  $x1$ = sum of skinfolds. $x2$ = age in years. Sites: chest, abdomen and thigh.
- Body density = $1.1125025 - 0.0013125(x1) + 0.0000055(x1)2 - 0.0000244(x2)$.
  $x1$ = sum of skinfolds. $x2$ = age in years. Sites: Chest, triceps, and subscapular.

Women
- Body density = $1.0994921 - 0.0009929(x3) + 0.0000023(x3)2 - 0.0001392(x4)$.
  $x3$ = sum of skinfolds. $x4$ = age in years. Sites: tricep, thigh and suprailium.
- Body density = $1.089733 - 0.0009245(x3) = 0.0000025(x3)2 - 0.0000979(x4)$.
  $x3$ = sum of skinfolds. $x4$ = age in years. Sites: triceps, suprailium and abdomen.

The most commonly used techniques concerning how to properly place the skinfold calipers on the six distinct sites used in the aforementioned sample equations generally adhere to the following guidelines:

Chest: diagonal fold halfway between the anterior axillary line (frontal portion of the armpit) and nipple for men and one third the distance from the anterior axillary line to the nipple for women.

Triceps: vertical fold taken in the middle of the back of the upper arm, halfway between the tip of the shoulder and tip of the elbow, elbow extended and relaxed.

Subscapular: fold taken on a diagonal line coming from the vertebral border 1-2 cm from the inferior angle of the scapula.

Abdominal: vertical fold taken at approximately one inch to the right of the umbilicus (belly button).

Suprailium: diagonal fold taken above the crest of the ilium (hip bone). The fold should follow the natural diagonal line of the hip at this point.

Thigh: vertical fold taken on the front thigh halfway between the hip and knee.

Once your level of body density has been identified, that calculation is then incorporated into an equation for determining percent body fat. Several such equations have been developed, including those devised by Brozek et al. (1963) and Siri (1961):

> • Brozek: Body fat % = 457/body density) - 414.2
> • Siri: Body fat % = (495/body density) = 45

Skinfold measurements have several advantages and disadvantages when used to assess body composition. Among the positive features of skinfold measurements are: they require little or no space to conduct the testing; they involve inexpensive equipment; the testing can be done quickly and easily; and the measures when obtained properly have a relatively high correlation with hydro-static weighing—the accepted "gold" standard. The major disadvantage to skinfold measuring is the potential for inaccurate measurements arising from measurements at the wrong sites, inconsistencies attendant to differences between the various types of calipers and the techniques employed by testors, and the inconsistency between the different equations used for estimating body density and percent body fat.

Other non-laboratory techniques commonly used for assessing body composition include: height-weight tables, relative weight (the ratio of actual weight to desirable weight), the body mass index, and circumference measurements. Although each method has the distinct advantage of being easy to administer, they all possess particular features which somewhat limit their usefulness.

CARDIORESPIRATORY FITNESS*

Cardiorespiratory (aerobic) fitness is considered by many experts to be the single most important component of physical fitness. In general, it is defined as the ability of your body to engage in relatively strenuous physical activity for an extended period of time. Dependent upon the combined efficiency of your lungs, heart, and circulatory system, cardiorespiratory fitness plays an essential role in sustained activities which involve the large muscle groups of your body. Your ability to sustain such activities is directly related to the capacity of your body to deliver oxygen to the working muscles. Because research has shown that indi-viduals who exercise regularly and are aerobically fit are less likely to suffer from any of the several serious "medical conditions" (e.g., atherosclerosis, hyperten-sion, angina, myocardial infarction, stroke, etc.), the need to accurately assess your level of cardiorespiratory fitness is critical.

---

* For normative data and relevant table relating to the assessment tests for cardiorespiratory fitness which are discussed this section, refer to *Exercise Physiology Laboratory Manual* by G.M. Adams; Dubuque, IA: Wm. C. Brown Publishers, 1990.

LABORATORY TESTS FOR CARDIORESPIRATORY FITNESS

Within a laboratory setting, cardiorespiratory fitness can be either directly measured or indirectly estimated. In turn, the indirect estimation of cardiorespiratory fitness can be based on your response to exercise involving either a maximal effort (on your part) or a submaximal effort.

Currently, most members of the exercise science and medical communities believe that the single most accurate means of assessing aerobic fitness is through a laboratory test which directly measures oxygen uptake during maximal exercise. This assessment technique is usually referred to as a maximal exercise (stress) test. The procedure requires several items: an exercise modality, such as a treadmill, a bicycle ergometer, or a stair climbing machine; a metabolic measuring system (to measure oxygen, carbon dioxide, and the volume of expired air); and an electrocardiogram to monitor the subject's heart activity and heart rate during the test. It also requires highly trained personnel to administer the test.

During a maximal exercise stress test, your physiological responses (heart rate, blood pressure, oxygen consumption, etc.) are periodically monitored as the test proceeds gradually from a relatively low-level exercise intensity to a maximal aerobic effort. The test is terminated when you reach a point of volitional fatigue (e.g., you can't continue exercising) or when your oxygen consumption levels off despite the fact that the intensity of the exercise keeps increasing. Your highest level of oxygen consumption is referred to as your maximal oxygen uptake ($\dot{V}O_2$ max).

The average male individual tends to have a $\dot{V}O_2$ max of 3-4 liters of oxygen per minute, while more highly trained endurance athletes have been observed to have an aerobic capacity of 5-6 liters per minute. Because aerobic capacity is related to body size, larger individuals tend to have higher scores. By factoring in body weight (dividing the maximal oxygen consumption value in liters by a subject's body weight expressed in kilograms), it becomes possible to compare the $\dot{V}O_2$ max of individuals—regardless of body weight. Table 10-1 provides norms

Table 10-1. Standards for Evaluating Cardiorespiratory (Aerobic) Fitness.

			$\dot{V}O_2$ MAX(METs) *				
AGE	LOW	FAIR	AVERAGE	GOOD	HIGH	ATHLETIC	OLYMPIC
WOMEN							
20-29	<8.0	8.3-9.7	10.0-12.3	12.6-13.7	14.0-15.1	15.4-16.8	17.1+
30-39	<7.7	8.0-9.4	9.7-11.7	12.0-13.4	13.7-14.8	15.1-16.6	16.8+
40-49	<7.1	7.4-8.8	9.1-11.4	11.7-12.8	13.1-14.3	14.6-16.0	16.3+
50-59	<6.0	6.3-7.7	8.0-10.3	10.6-11.7	12.0-12.8	13.1-14.0	14.3+
60-69	<4.8	5.1-6.3	6.6-8.8	9.1-10.3	10.6-11.4	11.7-12.6	12.8+
MEN							
20-29	<10.8	11.1-12.3	12.6-14.6	14.8-16.0	16.3-17.7	18.0-19.7	20.0+
30-39	<9.7	10.1-11.1	11.4-13.4	13.7-14.6	14.8-16.3	16.6-18.3	18.6+
40-49	<8.6	8.8-10.0	10.3-12.3	12.6-13.4	13.7-15.1	15.4-17.1	17.4+
50-59	<7.1	7.4-8.8	9.1-11.1	11.4-12.3	12.6-13.7	14.0-15.7	16.0+
60-69	<6.0	6.3-7.4	7.7-10.0	10.3-11.1	11.4-12.6	12.8-14.0	14.3+

* to convert METs to ml/kg/min., simply multiply by 3.5

for $\dot{V}O_2$ max to determine the aerobic fitness classification for an individual based on age and sex.

While direct analysis of expired gases yields the most accurate determination of $\dot{V}O_2$ max, such a method is—for the most part—not very feasible. It's simply too time-consuming, costly and complex to collect expired gases for this technique to be practical for most individuals. As a result, exercise scientists have developed equations for predicting $\dot{V}O_2$ max on the basis of your highest achieved workload or how long (time-wise) it takes you to reach a point of volitional fatigue while exercising rather than on the collection and analysis of expired gases. Similar to a $\dot{V}O_2$ max test, such a method also uses a graded exercise test. However, it does not involve the collection and analysis of expired gases.

Treadmill (Maximal Testing). A number of equations have been developed which employ the treadmill as the exercise modality for predicting $\dot{V}O_2$ max. Four of the most popular equations use either the Bruce, the Balke, or the Ellestad protocols. The following sample equations are grouped according to gender. The

---

- **Men: Cardiac and Healthy/Active (mean age = 48.1 ± 16.3 yrs).**
  Bruce Protocol: $\dot{V}O_2$ max(ml/kg/min) = 14.8 - 1.379(time) + 0.451(time^2) - 0.012(time^3). Time should be expressed in minutes and tenths of minutes.

- **Men: Active and Sedentary (mean age = 40.5 ± 5.3 yrs; range = 35-55 yrs old).**
  The Balke Protocol, which was employed to develop the equation for this group, uses a constant speed of 3.3mph and increases elevation 1% every minute. The initial work load is 3.3mph/0% for the first minute. The Ellestad test employed the following protocol: 1.7mph/10% for 2 min; 3/0mph/10% for 2 min; 4.0mph/10% for 2 min; 5.0mph/10% for 3 min; 6.0mph/15% for 2 min; 7.0mph/15% for 2 min; and 8.0mph/15% for 2 min.

  Balke Protocol: $\dot{V}O_2$ max (ml/kg/min) = 1.444 (time) + 14.99.
  Bruce Protocol: $\dot{V}O_2$ max (ml/kg/min) = 4.326 (time) - 4.66.
  Ellestad Protocol: $\dot{V}O_2$ max (ml/kg/min) = 3.933 (time) + 4.46.
  Time should be expressed in minutes and fractions of minutes for all these protocols.

- **Women: Healthy (mean age = 26.9 ± 5.2 yrs, range = 20-42 yrs).**
  The Balke Protocol used in this equation incorporates a constant speed of 3.0 mph. The initial work load is 3/0mph/0% and increases 2.5% every 3 minutes.

  Balke: $\dot{V}O_2$ max (ml/kg/min) = 0.023 (time in sec) + 5.2
  Bruce: $\dot{V}O_2$ max (ml/kg/min) = 0.073 (time in sec) - 3.9

- **Men and Women: Healthy/Active and Sedentary (men mean age = 48.6 ± 11.1 yrs; women mean age = 41.4 ± 11.2 yrs).**

  Bruce: $\dot{V}O_2$ max (ml/kg/min) = 6.70 = 2.82 (gender) + 0.056 (time in sec).
  Gender: 1 = men; 2 = women.

average age and the age range of the population used to develop the equations are also noted. All of the equations that are based on the Bruce Protocol employed the standard protocol which incorporates 3-minute stages as follows: 1.7mph/10% (elevation level); 2.5mph/12%; 3.4mph/14%; 4.2mph/16%; 5,0mph/20%; and 6.0mph/22%.

Cycle Ergometer (Maximal Testing). Cycle ergometers can also be used in maximal tests to predict $\dot{V}O_2$ max and estimate CR fitness. For the average person, a maximal cycle ergometer test is very difficult to perform. The great amount of localized muscular fatigue experienced during these kinds of incremental tests requires an individual to exhibit a relatively high degree of motivation to reach a true maximal work level. As a result, this type of testing has not been found to be preferable when a treadmill is available and the subject is fully ambulatory. Most cycling tests use a constant pedal rate (mechanically braked cycles) and require the work load to be increased until the subject reaches volitional fatigue. The stage duration can be 2-3 minutes in length, while work rate changes are typically 150-300 kgm/min (25-50 Watts), depending upon the fitness level of the individual.

The work rate increments on cycle ergometer testing are typically set at 150 kgm/min (25 Watts) for women, older adults, and unfit men; while increments of 300 kgm/min (50 Watts) are used for more trained individuals. The data used to predict $\dot{V}O_2$ max is the final work rate attained during the test. $\dot{V}O_2$ max is then estimated by means of the following equation (research suggests that the most accurate estimates are provided by achieved work rates which range between 300-1200 kgm/min or 50-200 Watts):

$$\dot{V}O_2 \text{ max (in ml/min)} = 2\,WR + 3.5\,BW$$
$$WR = \text{final work rate (in kgm/min)}$$
$$BW = \text{body weight in kilograms}$$

StairMaster® Exercise System (Maximal Testing). StairMaster exercise systems—models 5000 and 6000—have gained popularity as an effective means for maximal aerobic testing. The protocols for a StairMaster exercise system which have been reported in the literature involved initial step rates of 30-50 steps/min (approx. 4.5-6.0 METs) and mandated incremental increases in the step rate of 10-25/min (approx. 1-2 METs) every 2-3 minutes. Predicting $\dot{V}O_2$ max on your performance on a StairMaster exercise system is based on the final step rate you achieve during the test. The following equation can be used to predict $\dot{V}O_2$ max from maximal step rate:

$$\dot{V}O_2 \text{ max (ml/kg/min)} = 29.95 + .322 \text{ (max step rate - 85)}$$

$\dot{V}O_2$ max can also be predicted from exercise which does not involve a maximal effort. The primary advantage of using submaximal test data to predict $\dot{V}O_2$ max is that the intensity associated with a maximal effort is not required. Even though predicting $\dot{V}O_2$ max from submaximal testing is somewhat less accurate than predictions from maximal exercise data, it is a much safer process, particularly if response monitoring equipment is not available.

In general, submaximal laboratory setting assessments of $\dot{V}O_2$ max are based on your heart rate response to exercise. As a result, accurate heart rate measurements are absolutely essential when estimating $\dot{V}O_2$ max from submaximal protocols. It is recommended that either an electrocardiograph (when available) or a stethoscope be used to monitor heart rate. When neither tool is available (a somewhat common occurrence), palpation is used to detect and measure heart rate. It is strongly recommended, however, that individuals practice locating and counting their pulse rate during exercise prior to using this method during an actual test. The primary exercise modality for submaximal testing has traditionally been the cycle ergometer, although in some instances, treadmills and the StairMaster 4000PT* have been used.

Cycle Ergometer (Submaximal Testing). Submaximal cycle ergometer tests are popular assessment techniques for aerobic fitness. Perhaps the most commonly used submaximal cycle procedures are the YMCA protocol and the Astrand-Rhyming protocol. The YMCA protocol uses either two or three, three-minute stages of continuous exercise. The test is designed to raise the heart rate of the subject to between 110-150 beats/min for two consecutive stages. An important point to remember is that two consecutive heart rate measurements must be obtained in the 110-150 beats/min range to predict $\dot{V}O_2$ max. In the YMCA protocol, each work load is administered for three minutes, with heart rates recorded during the final 15-30 seconds of both the second and third minutes. If these heart rates are not within five beats/min of each other, then the current work load should be extended for an additional minute. The heart rate measured during the last minute of each stage is plotted against work load as described on the worksheet illustrated in Figure 10-1. The line generated from the plotted points is then extended to the age-predicted maximal heart rate. A corresponding maximal work load and $\dot{V}O_2$ max can then be estimated.

The Astrand-Rhyming cycle ergometer test is a single work load test of six minutes duration. The suggested work load is selected based upon gender and an individual's activity status as follows: males—unconditioned, 300 or 600 kgm/min (50 or 100 Watts), or conditioned, 600 or 900 kgm/min (100 or 150 Watts); females—unconditioned, 300 or 450 kgm/min (50 or 75 Watts), or conditioned, 450 or 600 kpm/min (75 or 100 Watts). The pedal rate is set at 50 rpm. Heart rate is measured during the 5th and 6th minutes of work. The average heart rate is then used to estimate $\dot{V}O_2$ max from a nomogram or a table of normative values which might be corrected for age.

---

* Editors' Note: A submaximal exercise testing protocol for use with the StairMaster® 4000PT® has recently been developed and is currently being validated. It can be obtained upon request from the Department of Sports Medicine, StairMaster® Sports/Medical Products, Inc., 12421 Willows Rd. N.E., Kirkland, Washington 98034.

Figure 10-1. Worksheet for determining $\dot{V}O_2$ max from submaximal heart rates obtained during the YMCA's submaximal cycle test.

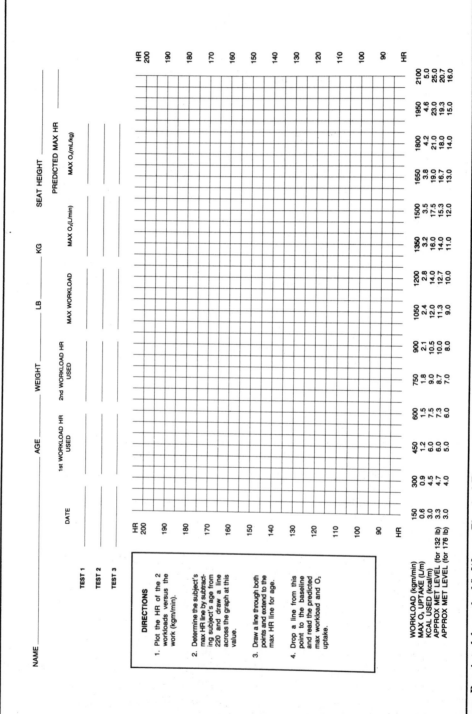

Source: Reprinted from the Y's Way to Physical Fitness (3rd Ed. Champaign, IL, Human Kinetics Publishers, 1989), with permission of the YMCA of the U.S.A., 101 N. Wacker Drive, Chicago, IL 60606.

NON-LABORATORY TESTS FOR CARDIORESPIRATORY FITNESS

Your aerobic fitness level can also be predicted by tests which do not have to be performed in a laboratory setting. In general, while such methods are not as accurate as most laboratory tests, they are relatively easy to administer. In addition, they have the advantage of requiring almost no equipment and being able to be performed almost anywhere. Two of the most popular types of non-laboratory tests for assessing cardiorespiratory fitness are performance (field) tests and step tests.

Depending on the specific performance test, you try to run/walk a certain distance as fast as you can or you see how far you can run/walk with a specific time limit. Such tests appear to be particularly well suited to healthy, active individuals who are highly motivated and able to pace themselves for the specified distance or time. Field tests are also useful when large numbers of people are to be tested. These tests require the use of well marked, level terrain (preferably a track) to easily measure the total distance travelled and an accurate timing device (a stopwatch or a digital watch).

The potential downside of performance tests is that because they encourage you to exert a maximal effort, they can involve some degree of risk. Make sure that if you experience extreme fatigue, dizziness, nausea or chest pain while taking a performance test, that you stop the test immediately. Once you've improved your aerobic fitness level through a gradual (sound) aerobic exercise program, you can then retake the test.

Two of the most commonly employed performance tests are the 1.5-mile run for time and the 12-minute walk-run test for distance. The objective in the 1.5-mile test is to cover the distance in as short a time as possible and, in the case of the 12-minute walk-run test, to cover the greatest distance in the allotted time period. The results of each test are then compared to a table of age and gender-related normative standards to provide an estimate or the cardiorespiratory fitness level of the individual being tested.

In the past few years, a one-mile walking test (Rockport Fitness Walking Test) has gained popularity as an effective means for estimating cardiorespiratory fitness. The objective of this test is to walk one mile as fast as possible, preferably on a track or level surface. Your heart rate is recorded immediately at the end of the walk and is used as a predictor variable for $\dot{V}O_2$ max. Your time in completing the test is then entered into the following equation:

$$\dot{V}O_2 \text{ max (ml/kg/min)} = 132.853 - (0.0769 \times BW) - (0.3877 \times A) + (6.315 \times G) - (3.2649 \times T) - (0.1565 \times HR).$$ BW = body weight in pounds; A = age in years; G = gender: 0 = female, 1 = male; T = time for the walk in minutes and hundreths of a minutes; HR = heart rate taken at the end of the one-mile walk expressed in beats per minute.

Similar to performance tests, step tests also permit many people to be evaluated at the same time. As a general rule, such tests only require minimal and inexpensive equipment to conduct. All that is necessary to administer a step test is a bench/step of an appropriate height for the desired test, a metronome to set the cadence and an accurate watch or stopwatch.

In a step test, you step up and down on a bench (of a prescribed height—usually between 8-20 inches) while alternating feet, at a predetermined rate (usually 20 to 30 steps per minute), for a predetermined period of time (usually five minutes or so). Following your exercise bout, your pulse is taken at designated intervals (usually 15-second to 30-second intervals). When you stop exercising, your heart rate decreases rapidly in the first minute. After the first minute, the decline in heart rate becomes much more gradual. The faster your heart rate returns to normal, the more aerobically fit you are. Your heart rate response at a certain postexercise point can then either be plugged into a prediction equation to estimate $\dot{V}O_2$ max, or used to compare against normative data tables (which have been adjusted for age, weight and gender) to show you how you stack up relatively speaking against other individuals. The simplicity and ease of scoring a step test make it widely applicable to a wide variety of situations and needs.

While a number of different step tests have been developed over the years, two of the most widely used procedures are the Queen's College Step Test and the Forestry Step Test. Both techniques employ recovery heart rates to estimate $\dot{V}O_2$ max. The Queen's College Test requires that you step up and down on a bench or bleacher which is approximately 16.25 inches high for three minutes. The cadence is set with a metronome at 22 steps/min (88 on the metronome) for women and 24 steps/min (96 on the metronome) for men. At the end of the test, your standing heart rate is taken continuously beginning five seconds into the recovery time for the next 15 seconds (i.e., 5-20 sec of recovery). The measured heart rate should then be multiplied by four and entered into the appropriate equation*:

> Men: $\dot{V}O_2$ max = 111.33 - (0.42 x step-test heart rate)
> Women: $\dot{V}O_2$ max = 65.81 - (0.1847 x step-test heart rate)

The Forestry Step Test was developed in 1977 as a modification of the Astrand-Rhyming protocol. It appears to have wider applicability than the Queen's College Test in that age-adjusted norms are provided. This test requires that you step up and down for five minutes at 22.5 steps/min (90 on the metronome). The step height is set at 40 cm (15.75 inches) for men and 33 cm (13 inches) for women. At the end of the five minute test, you are required to sit down, whereupon your heart rate is measured, beginning 15 seconds into the recovery, for 15 seconds (i.e., time 15-30 seconds during recovery). Your pulse count (the actual count, not the one-minute heart rate) is then matched with your weight and compared with age-adjusted normative data. This comparison then yields a value

---

*Note: Both equations estimate $\dot{V}O_2$ max expressed in ml/kg/min and are applicable when testing college-age men and women.

which reflects your estimated $\dot{V}O_2$ max (expressed in ml/kg/min). This value can subsequently be used to identify your relative CR level by comparing it to existing norms for $\dot{V}O_2$ max.

If you decide to assess your aerobic fitness level with a step test, you should keep in mind that one of the main disadvantages of using a step test—particularly for older individuals or for those who are in relatively poor condition—is the potential for tripping. Such an occurrence may be more likely during the Forestry Step Test, since this test requires you to exercise for a longer duration than does the Queen's College Test. Ensuring that you have something to lean on if necessary, such as a handrail, the back of a chair, or a partner, may help you to relax and provide an added degree of safety during the step test. You should keep in mind, however, that these techniques will reduce the actual amount of work you perform.

ASSESSING MUSCULAR FITNESS

In general, muscular fitness is defined as the capacity of your muscles to "do what you need them to do when you need it to be done." Given the role that your muscular system plays in enabling you to perform the basic tasks of daily living, to avoid undue risk of being injured, and to participate in leisure-oriented physical activities, the importance of muscular fitness cannot be overemphasized.

Most exercise scientists contend that muscular fitness collectively should be viewed as being comprised of two distinct components of physical fitness: muscular strength and muscular endurance. *Muscular strength* can be defined as the ability of a muscle or a muscle group to exert maximum force. Muscular *endurance*, on the other hand, can be defined as the ability of a muscle or a muscle group to exert submaximal force for an extended period of time. Accordingly, the first step in assessing muscular fitness involves identifying which muscle-related component of physical fitness you wish to measure—muscular strength or muscular endurance.

Regardless of which component of muscular fitness is to be tested, a number of factors* must be taken into consideration, including:

1. *The devices commonly employed to assess muscular fitness all have design features and usage requirements that make the test results less than 100% reliable.* For example, if the device has a pad on it that you push against, the extent to which you depress the pad will effect the measurement obtained. By the same token, if the procedures for using the device require that your body must be in an exact angular position, it can be very

---

* Author's Note: Much of this discussion concerning the potential problems involved with muscular fitness testing is based on information presented in *Advanced Fitness Assessment and Exercise Prescription*, (Vivian H. Heyward); pp. 114-116; used with the permission of the publisher, Human Kinetics Publishers.

difficult to assume a position that mandates a particular joint angle each and every time you are tested. Both examples serve to confirm the fact that measuring muscular fitness is not a process that involves unequivocal precision. As a result, knowing the design limitations of the device you are using in the assessment process, as well as the potential problems that might occur with any deviation in the protocol for using the device, will enable you to be better prepared to interpret the results that are obtained.

2. *Muscular strength and muscular endurance are specific to the muscle or muscle group, the type of muscular contraction (static or dynamic—concentric, eccentric, isokinetic), the speed of muscular contraction (slow or fast), and the joint angle being tested (static contraction).* Accordingly, the results of any one test are specific to the specific parameters of the procedure used to obtain the measurement. No single test exists for evaluating total body muscular strength or muscular endurance.

3. *The test items used to measure either muscular strength or muscular endurance should be selected with care.* Assessment batteries which are designed to measure muscular strength should not include maximum repetition tests. By the same token, the most appropriate tests for measuring muscular endurance are those which are proportional to the body weight or the maximum strength level of the individual being tested.

4. *Because muscular fitness is often directly related to both the total body weight and the amount of lean muscle mass of the individual being tested, the test results should be expressed in relative terms.* The value of expressing muscular fitness test results in relative terms is particularly worthwhile when comparing one individual to another or one group to another.

5. *Because most muscular fitness tests require a maximum effort by the individual being tested, (as much as possible) care should be taken to control those factors that might affect maximum performance.* Among the factors that could influence how well an individual performs are: time of day, sleep, medication, motivation level, energy level, and emotional state. Steps should also be undertaken to ensure that the maximal effort being exerted does not subject the individual to an undue level of exertion.

6. Caution *should be taken when comparing the results of the muscular fitness testing to normative data.* Much of the normative data relating to muscular fitness is either out-dated or, to a degree, invalid or unreliable.*

Muscular fitness is typically assessed using either tests that employ specific devices for measuring muscular strength and muscular endurance or calisthenic-

---

* Editors' Note: A critical need exists for additional normative data for both muscular strength and muscular endurance. Compared to the other basic components of physical fitness, the two muscle-related components have received relatively minimal attention by the exercise science community.

type tests. Most of the testing (but not all) that employs devices is conducted in a laboratory rather than a field setting because the devices often require trained personnel to use and are relatively expensive. Calisthenic-type tests, on the other hand, can be performed in a non-laboratory setting. This type of testing usually requires little or no equipment, can be performed almost anywhere, enables more than one person to be tested at the same time, and involves bodily movements which are somewhat more functional in nature.

TESTS INVOLVING DEVICES FOR MEASURING MUSCULAR FITNESS

A number of devices for measuring muscular fitness have been developed, including dynamometers, cable tensiometers, electromechanical and hydraulic devices, and resistance machines. Deciding which (if any) device to use can involve several factors, including the cost and availability of the apparatus, the level of expertise required to use the device, the muscle or muscle group to be tested, the type of information desired, and for what purpose the findings will be used.*

CALISTHENIC-TYPE TESTS FOR MEASURING MUSCULAR FITNESS

In certain situations, calisthenic-type tests may be a more appropriate means for assessing muscular fitness. Calisthenic-type tests involve measuring in terms specific to the muscle-related component being assessed how (quantitatively) well you can perform calisthenic-type exercises (e.g., push-ups, chin-ups, pull-ups, dips, sit-ups, etc.) When you measure dynamic muscular strength by a calisthenic-type test, you determine the maximum amount of weight that you can lift in excess of your body weight for one repetition of the (exercise) movement. On the other hand, assessing dynamic muscular endurance through the use of a calisthenic-type tests involves determining the maximum number of repetitions of each (calisthenic-type) exercise you can perform. Because calisthenic-type testing for muscular endurance is quite popular with several organizations (e.g., the U.S. military, the President's Council on Physical Fitness, etc.), considerable normative data relating to the results from this type of testing exists.

ASSESSING FLEXIBILITY

Flexibility is generally defined as the ability of a skeletal joint to move fluidly through its full range of motion (ROM). Range of motion is highly specific to the joint and depends on the joint structure. Flexibility in one specific joint does not necessarily indicate flexibility in other joints. For example, triaxial joints (e.g., hip, shoulder) afford a greater degree of movement in more directions than either uniaxial (e.g., knee, elbow) or biaxial (e.g., wrist) joints.

Accordingly, no general flexibility test exists for total body flexibility.

---

* Author's Note: For more information refer to chapter 5 for a comprehensive overview of the devices most commonly employed to measure muscular fitness.

Specific to each joint, your level of flexibility is affected by several factors, including age, gender, and the type and amount of physical activity in which you are involved.

Flexibility can be either static or dynamic. Static flexibility is a measure of the overall ROM at a specific joint; dynamic flexibility, on the other hand, is a measure of the amount of resistance to movement by the joint. Both types of flexibility play significant roles in physical activity. Despite the fact that assessing joint stiffness and resistance to movement (dynamic flexibility) may be more meaningful than absolute ROM data, relatively little research has been conducted to assess dynamic flexibility.

Several techniques—both laboratory and field—have been developed to assess static flexibility. Traditionally, static flexibility is measured by determining ROM either directly or indirectly.

DIRECT METHODS FOR MEASURING STATIC FLEXIBILITY

Static flexibility can be measured directly through the use of a device specifically designed to measure ROM, such as a goniometer, an electrogoniometer, and a Leighton flexometer. Such tools are typically used in laboratory or clinical settings under very controlled conditions.

A goniometer is a protractor-like instrument with two steel (or Plexiglas) arms that enable you to measure angles. The difference between the joint angles (in degrees) which are measured at the extremes of a movement is the ROM. An electrogoniometer is a device that allows you to assess ROM (joint angles) by means of electrical input. The Leighton flexometer is a device which consists of a weighted 360-degree dial and a weighted pointer. The ROM for a specific skeletal joint is measured in relation to the downward pull of gravity on the dial and the pointer. After you perform a movement, the pointer is locked in at the extreme ROM you achieved, which enables you to read the degree of arc through which the movement occurred directly from the dial.

INDIRECT METHODS FOR MEASURING STATIC FLEXIBILITY

Static flexibility can be assessed indirectly through linear measurements of the ROM. Among the examples of field tests which are commonly used for such purposes are: the sit-and-reach test, the modified sit-and-reach test, the shoulder rotation test, the ankle flexion test, the ankle extension test, the shoulder-and-wrist elevation test, and the trunk-and-neck extension test. Field tests are specific to the joints involved in the movement, measure to the nearest 1/4 inch how far you can either extend or flex during a specific movement, and usually require three trial performances—the best of which is counted.*

---

*Refer to *Practical Measurements for Evaluation in Physical Education* (4th Edition), by Barry L. Johnson and Jack K. Nelson (Macmillan Publishing Company), for a detailed explanation of the protocol for performing specific field tests for assessing flexibility.

THE CRITICAL FIRST STEP

A strong argument can be made that the initial step in the process for developing an appropriate fitness program for you *MUST BE TO EVALUATE YOUR EXISTING LEVEL OF FITNESS*. Properly assessing the status of the various components of physical fitness will facilitate the likelihood that you be able to attain the full benefits of a physically active lifestyle. Knowing how fit you are enables you to be better prepared to identify and take the appropriate steps for developing the level of fitness you want, need, and deserve. ❏

BIBLIOGRAPHY •

1. American College of Sports Medicine. Guidelines for Exercise Testing and Prescription, 4th Ed. Philadelphia, PA: Lea and Febiger, 1991.
2. American Heart Association. Exercise and Training of Apparently *Healthy Individuals: A Handbook for Physicians*. Dallas, TX: American Heart Association, 1972.
3. Astrand, I. "A method for prediction of aerobic work capacity for females and males of different ages." *Acta Physiol Scand* 49(Suppl.):S43-S60, 1960.
4. Astrand, P.O., Rodahl, K. *Textbook of Work Physiology*, 3rd Ed. New York, NY: McGraw-Hill, 1986.
5. Ben-Ezra, V., Verstraete, R. "Stair climbing: An alternative exercise modality for firefighters." *J Occup Med* 30:103-105, 1988.
6. Brozek, J., Grande, F., Anderson, J., et al. "Densitometric analysis of body composition: Revision of some quantitative assumptions." *Ann NY Acad Sci* 110:113-140, 1963.
7. Carroll, K., Marshall, D., Sockler, J., et al. "An equation for predicting maximal oxygen consumption on the StairMaster." *Med Sci Sports Exerc* 22(2):S11, 1990.
8. Foster, C., Jackson, A.S., Pollock, M.L., et al. "Generalized equations for predicting functional capacity from treadmill performance." *Am Heart J* 107:1229-1234, 1984.
9. Golding, L.A., Myers, C.F., Sinning, W.E. *The Y's Way to Physical Fitness, Revised*. Chicago, IL: National Board of YMCA, 1982.
10. Heyward, V.H. *Advanced fitness assessment & exercise prescription*, 2nd Ed. Champaign, IL: Human Kinetics Publishers, 1991.
11. Holland, G.J., Weber, F., Heng, et al. "Maximal steptreadmill exercise and treadmill exercise by patients with coronary heart disease: A comparison." *J Cardiopulmonary Rehabil* 8:58-68, 1988.
12. Jackson, A.S., Pollock, M.L. "Generalized equations for predicting body density of men." *Brit J Nutr* 40:497-504, 1978.
13. Jackson, A.S., Pollock, M.L., Ward, A. "Generalized equations for predicting body density of women." *Med Sci Sports Exerc* 12:175-182, 1980.
14. Jackson, A.S., Pollock, M.L. "Practical assessment of body composition." *Phys Sportsmed* 13(5):76-90, 1985.
15. Kline, G.M., Porci, J.P., Hintermeister, R., et al. "Estimation of VO_2 max from a one-mile track walk, gender, age, and body weight." *Med Sci Sports Exerc* 19(3):253-259, 1987.
16. Leighton, J. "Instrument and technique for measurement of range of joint motion." *Arch Phys Med Rehabil* 36:571-578, 1955.
17. McArdle, W.D., Katch, F.I., Pechar, G.S., et al. "Reliability and interrelationships between maximal oxygen intake, physical work capacity and step-test scores in college women." *Med Sci Sports* 4:182-186, 1972.

18. Nieman, D.C. *Fitness and Sports Medicine: An Introduction*, 2nd Ed. Palo Alto, CA: Bull Publishing Company, 1990.
19. Pollock, M.L., Foster, C., Schmidt, D., et al. "Comparative analysis of physiologic responses to three different maximal graded exercise test protocols in healthy women." *Am Heart J* 103:363-373, 1982.
20. Sharkey, B.J. *Physiology of Fitness*, 2nd Ed. Champaign, IL: Human Kinetics Publishers, Inc., 1984.
21. Siri, W.E. "Body composition from fluid spaces and density." *In* Brozek, J., Henschel, A., (Eds), *Techniques for Measuring Body Composition*. Washington, DC: National Academy of Sciences, 1961.

CHAPTER 11

● ●

DEVELOPING A PERSONALIZED EXERCISE PROGRAM: PRESCRIPTION GUIDELINES

by

Gerald D. Thompson, M.S.
and
B. Don Franks, Ph.D.

● ● ●

"My present prescription for exercise is as follows: Daily
—at least 60 minutes of physical activity, not necessarily
vigorous, nor all at the same time. Weekly—at least two
or three periods of 30 minutes of intermittent or sustained
activity at a submaximal rate of work are necessary for
maintaining good cardiovascular fitness."
                                                    Dr. Per-Olof Astrand

*I*n general, the statement made by Dr. Astrand concerning what constitutes
a sufficient quantity of exercise for maintaining personal fitness is supported by
the American College of Sports Medicine (ACSM) and prevailing exercise science
research. His statement, however, needs some qualification and further quantification. An exercise prescription is a personalized program of recommended
physical activity which is designed to enhance, maintain, or restore positive health
and fitness. Specific guidelines for the intensity, duration, frequency, type, and
progression of exercise are integral components of a sound exercise prescription.

An individual's health and fitness status, the exercise setting, the program
goals, and the participant's goals are critical factors in the development of an
exercise prescription. As a general rule, exercise prescriptions are either self-
developed or designed by professionally trained personnel who are employed at
health-fitness facilities. Regardless of what option is followed, the prescription

must be based on the aforementioned factors. Health-Fitness facilities usually administer some type of Health Status Questionnaire (refer to Figures 2-1 and 2-2) to gather information on those factors to decide which activities (as outlined by criteria established by the ACSM) will be most appropriate to include in an individual's initial exercise program. Finally, it should be noted that once an exercise program has actually begun, periodic evaluations of an individual's health and fitness status need to be conducted to assess the individual's adaptation to the exercise regime and whether or not adjustments in the program's protocol should be undertaken.

If you are engaging in a "self-administered" exercise program and are charged with conducting your own periodic assessments of your personal level of fitness, you need to ensure that your efforts are based on sound information and techniques. If, however, you are one of the more than ten million Americans who belong to a health-fitness facility, the professional staff at that facility—in all likelihood—will include periodic evaluations of your health status and fitness progress as part of their efforts to serve you. In fact, the ACSM—in its recently developed "Consumer Guidelines for Selecting a Health-Fitness Facility," recommends that if you are considering becoming a member of a health-fitness club, you examine the policies of that facility with regard to medical clearance and personal fitness assessment before you join. In general, a health-fitness facility should adhere to the following fundamental policies:

- Recommends routine medical checkups and health screening as part of its standard operating procedures.
- Recommends low-intensity exercise (40 to 60% of maximal heart rate reserve) initially, for all apparently healthy individuals who display no unusual physiological signs or symptoms.
- Requires medical clearance before moderate or high-intensity exercise participation for individuals with:
  - known health problems, two or more major coronary risk factors, or signs or symptoms indicative of potential health problems (individuals at higher risk) refer to Tables 2-1 and 2-2, or
  - intentions of engaging in very strenuous activities (in athletic performance where the level of intensity is much higher than that needed for fitness gains).
- Recommends maximal graded exercise (stress) test (GXT), with physician's interpretation of ECG, prior to exercise participation for individuals with known cardiovascular disease, symptoms related to cardiovascular disease, significant risk factors for cardiovascular disease, and men over 40 years of age or women over 50 years of age.

The primary focus of this chapter is to provide an overview regarding factors that should be considered in developing fitness programs for apparently healthy adults. The apparently healthy population is generally characterized as being both symptom free and engaging in relatively routine physical activity. They can begin low intensity exercise programs without the need for exercise testing or medical examination as long as the exercise program progresses gradually and the individual is alert to the development of any unusual signs or symptoms. A simple, brief questionnaire called the Physical Activity Readiness Questionnaire (PAR-Q) has been found to be a valid screening instrument for both submaximal exercise testing and for beginning low-intensity and gently progressive (but not heavy or overly challenging) exercise programs (refer to Figure 2-1). Moderate-intensity exercise (60 to 80% $\dot{V}O_2$ max) is sufficiently intense to represent a substantial challenge to an individual because it will elicit significant increases in specific physiologic responses (e.g., heart rate and respiration). At or above age 40 in men, or age 50 in women, it is desirable for individuals to have both a medical examination and a supervised maximal exercise test before beginning a vigorous exercise program (refer to Table 2-3 for a summary of the basic guidelines for exercise testing and participation).

CARDIORESPIRATORY CONDITIONING

Based on the existing scientific evidence concerning exercise prescription for healthy adults and the need for such guidelines, the American College of Sports Medicine developed a position paper on exercise prescription which included the following recommendations concerning the quantity and quality of (exercise) training for developing and maintaining cardiorespiratory fitness and desirable body composition in a healthy adult.

1. Frequency of training: 3 to 5 days per week.

2. Intensity: 50% to 85% of maximum oxygen uptake $\dot{V}O_2$ max), 50% to 85% of maximum heart rate reserve, or 60% - 90% of maximal heart rate. It should be noted that exercise of low and moderate intensity may provide important health benefits and may result in increased fitness in some persons (e.g., those who were previously sedentary and low fit).

3. Duration of training: 20 to 60 minutes of continuous aerobic activity. The actual length of time you should exercise aerobically is generally dependent on the relative intensity level of the activity. For example, activities involving a lower intensity should be conducted over a longer period of time. Your emphasis should be placed on the total work you perform. Total work can be estimated by the caloric expenditure associated with the activity—a subject which will be discussed later in this chapter.

4. Mode of activity: An appropriate modality for developing cardiorespiratory fitness is any activity that uses the large muscle groups, that can be maintained continuously, and is rhythmical and aerobic in nature (e.g., running, jogging, walking, machine-based stair climbing, swimming, skating, bicycling, rowing, cross-country skiing, and various endurance game activities). Note: At the beginning of an exercise program, activities such as walking, jogging, machine-based stair climbing, and cycling are most recommended.

5. Rate of progression: In most instances, the ability of the body to adapt to the stresses imposed upon it (sometimes referred to as the training effect) allows individuals to gradually increase the total work they do over time. In continuous exercise, increasing the work performed can be achieved by increasing the intensity of the exercise, the duration of the exercise bout, or by some combination of the two. The most significant conditioning effects are typically observed during the first six to eight weeks of an exercise program. An individual's exercise prescription is normally adjusted as these conditioning effects occur. The extent of the adjustment depends on the individual involved, additional feedback from assessment efforts, and/or the exercise performance of the individual during exercise sessions.

DEVELOPING AN APPROPRIATE EXERCISE PRESCRIPTION

It should be noted that desirable outcomes can be attained with exercise programs that vary considerably in terms of mode, frequency, duration, and intensity. In addition, it should be remembered that some individuals achieve a faster (or greater) rate of improvement than others.

For example, if you have been relatively sedentary for years, you should expect to progress more slowly. In this instance, you should begin exercising at a level that you can easily complete and should then gradually increase the amount of work that you perform during a workout. On the other hand, if you are an individual who has been somewhat active, you may progress more rapidly in your exercise programs than a sedentary individual whose slower progression is necessary primarily to reduce injury potential and to assure appropriate adaptation in previously unused muscles. Finally, depending how your body responds (and adapts) to the demands imposed upon it by your exercise program, you need to be both willing and able to modify your exercise prescription as appropriate.

WARM-UP AND COOL-DOWN PHASES

Warm-up and cool-down activities should be an essential part of all exercise programs. The purpose of the warm-up is to prepare your body, especially your cardiovascular and musculoskeletal systems, for the conditioning or stimulus phase of the exercise session. The cool-down phase assures that venous return to your heart is maintained in the face of significant amounts of blood going to previously working muscles. Light aerobic endurance activities, coupled with stretching activities, provide the recommended basis for both the warm-up and cool-down phases.

The length of the warm-up and cool-down periods depends on several factors, including the type of activity engaged in during the conditioning period, the level of intensity of those activities, as well as the age and fitness level of the participant. In general, the warm-up and cool-down phases last approximately five to ten minutes each. If the time you have available to work out is less than usual, it is recommended that you reduce the time allotted for the conditioning phase of your workout, while retaining sufficient time for the warm-up and cool-down phases.

CARDIORESPIRATORY ENDURANCE ACTIVITIES

The ACSM differentiates between several types of cardiorespiratory endurance activities. Activities like walking, jogging, machine-based stair climbing, or cycling (referred to as Group 1 activities) can be easily maintained at a constant level of intensity. The variability between subjects in terms of energy expenditure is relatively low in these types of activities. In Group 2 activities, such as swimming or cross-country skiing, the rate of energy expenditure is highly related to skill. Although the level of intensity involved in Group 2 activities tends to vary between individuals, a relatively constant level of intensity can be maintained within a given individual. Tennis, basketball, and racquetball (referred to as Group 3 activities) by their very nature are highly variable in intensity both between individuals and within a specific individual.

The type of activities (Group 1, 2, or 3) prescribed for you will be highly dependent upon the results of your health risk appraisal assessment and your current fitness level. For example, Group 3 activities are generally not prescribed for unfit, at risk, or diseased individuals, because such activities can vary a great deal in their intensity.

INTENSITY OF EXERCISE

Perhaps the most important component of an exercise prescription is the level of exercise intensity. The prescribed level of intensity must be sufficient to overload the cardiovascular system, but not so severe that it overtaxes the system. For the apparently healthy individual who wants to develop and maintain cardiorespiratory fitness, the American College of Sports Medicine recommends that the intensity level of the exercise needs to be between 50 to 85 percent of the person's maximum oxygen uptake capacity ($\dot{V}O_2$ max). Exercise intensities between 60% to 80% of $\dot{V}O_2$ max are prescribed for most participants. It is generally believed, however, that the intensity threshold for a training effect is at the low end of this continuum for those who have been sedentary, and at the high end of the scale for those who are physically active.

CALCULATING EXERCISE INTENSITY

Exercise intensity can be prescribed in terms of heart rate (HR) by using specific heart rate values that are approximately equal to 60 to 80% of $\dot{V}O_2$ max. One method involves monitoring HR at each stage of a maximal graded exercise test (GXT). The HR is plotted on a graph against the $\dot{V}O_2$ (or MET) equivalents of each stage of the test in order to define the slope of the heart rate response to exercise.

From this relationship the exercise heart rate associated with a given percent of $\dot{V}O_2$ max can be obtained. While such a method is generally preferred, it does require a participant to complete a maximal GXT—with its associated logistical and safety considerations. Another method for assessing exercise intensity is based on the observation that 70 and 85% of maximal heart rate is equal to approximately 60 and 80% of functional capacity ($\dot{V}O_2$ max). For example:

> THR range = maximal HR x 0.70 and 0.85
> where:
> THR = training heart rate
> maximal HR = 220 - age (in years)

The third method for determining the exercise heart rate for training is to calculate the heart rate reserve (HRR). The HRR method of determining the training or target heart rate range, made popular by Karvonen, requires a few simple calculations:

> First, subtract resting HR from maximal HR to obtain HR reserve.
> Then, take 60% and 80% of the HR reserve.
> Then, add each value to resting HR to obtain the THR range.
>
> • THR range = [(maximal HR - resting HR) x 0.60 and 0.80] + resting HR[*]

Whenever possible, use an accurate measurement of maximal heart rate rather than a predicted or estimated one. Estimated maximum heart rates have the distinct disadvantage in that they are based on population averages, and, as a result, have a standard deviation of plus or minus 10-12 bpm.

Another method for prescribing and monitoring exercise intensity involves using ratings of perceived exertion (RPE—refer to Table 11-1). This method, developed by Swedish psychologist Gunnar Borg, uses a 15-point numerical scale ranging from 6 to 20 with the individual who is exercising providing a verbal description of how (relatively) difficult the exercise is based on categories assigned to every odd number. A perceived exertion rating of 12 to 13 has been shown to correspond to approximately 60% of $\dot{V}O_2$ max. A rating of 16 corresponds to approximately 80 to 85% of $\dot{V}O_2$ max. Therefore, an RPE range of 12 (somewhat hard) to 16 (hard) is recommended for most healthy adults.

Participants skilled at using RPE as an indicator of overall feeling of exertion can use it to specify an RPE level for conditioning. It can also be used in conjunction with a THR prescription. In addition, RPE can be used to modify an exercise prescription. RPE, for example, is often one of the first readily recognizable measures of (positive) changes in cardiorespiratory fitness.

---

[*] Resting HR is best determined while in a seated position immediately upon waking in the morning.

Table 11-1. The 15-point and 10-point Borg RPE scales.

Category (15-point) RPE Scale		Category/Ratio (10-point) RPE Scale	
6		0	Nothing at all
7	Very, very light	0.5	Very, very weak
8		1	Very weak
9	Very light	2	Weak
10		3	Moderate
11	Fairly light	4	Somewhat strong
12		5	Strong
13	Somewhat hard	6	
14		7	Very strong
15	Hard	8	
16		9	
17	Very hard	10	Very, very strong
18		*	Maximal
19	Very, very hard		
20			

From Noble, B.J., et al. *Med Sci Sports Exerc* 15:523-528, 1983.

DURATION OF THE EXERCISE SESSION

The duration of exercise refers to the amount of time (in minutes) that the proper intensity level should be maintained. Typically, a conditioning phase lasts for at least 20 to 30 minutes, which corresponds to the amount of time required for the improvement or maintenance of functional capacity. Individuals just beginning an exercise program should start with approximately 10-20 minutes of aerobic activity. On the other hand, individuals in average shape can exercise for a longer period of time (e.g., 20-30 minutes). Keep in mind that the optimum duration of an exercise session usually depends on the intensity level of the workout. More importantly, in order to achieve health and fitness benefits, exercise should be long enough to expend about 300 kcal.

FREQUENCY OF EXERCISE SESSION

Frequency of exercise refers to the number of exercise sessions per week. While some studies have been able to demonstrate improvements in cardiorespiratory fitness with an exercise frequency of less than three days per week, such improvements have tended to be minimal. It appears that the body responds best to three to five days per week of moderate-intensity aerobic exercise with sessions lasting 20-30 minutes. The traditional recommendation of a "work-one-day and rest-one-day" routine remains a valid approach if you want to improve your level of cardiorespiratory fitness. It should be pointed out that for previously sedentary individuals, the frequency level of your exercise program should initially be established at three days per week. More sessions would place them at undue risk for orthopedic injuries and expose them to an exercise environment which might have a negative effect on their level of exercise adherence. Individuals who desire to increase their frequency of training should gradually do so, depending on their age, initial and existing fitness status, and their personal needs, interests, and exercise objectives.

MODE OF EXERCISE

Activities should be selected on the basis of individual functional capacity, interest, time, personal goals, and objectives. A fitness program usually starts with activities quantifiable, such as walking, exercise cycling, or stair climbing, so that the proper exercise intensity which is appropriate for you can be determined and achieved. When you can exercise 3-4 days a week 30-40 minutes a day at that level, any activity utilizing large muscle groups can be incorporated into your exercise program.

RATE OF PROGRESSION

The recommended rate of progression in your exercise program depends on several interrelated factors, including your fitness status, health status, age, needs or goals, and support provided by friends and family. The American College of Sports Medicine defines three distinct stages of an exercise prescription.

1. Initial Conditioning Stage: This stage typically lasts 4-6 weeks, but may be longer depending on the participant's adaptation to the exercise program. ACSM suggests that you exercise at a level of intensity which is approximately 1 MET* lower than the one corresponding to an estimate of 40 to 85% (or lower than 50 to 90% of maximal heart rate) of your functional capacity in order to avoid undue muscle soreness, injury, discomfort, and discouragement.

2. Improvement Conditioning Stage: This stage lasts 12-20 weeks, and is the period during which progression is most rapid. The intensity level is increased to 50 to 85% of VO_2 max (60 to 90% of maximal heart rate), while the duration of the exercise session is increased as frequently as every two to three weeks. The frequency and magnitude of increments are dictated by the rate at which you adapt to the conditioning program.

3. Maintenance Conditioning Stage: When the desired level of conditioning is attained, the maintenance stage begins—usually after the first six months of training. At this time, the emphasis is often refocused from an exercise program involving primarily fitness activities to one which includes a more diverse array of enjoyable (lifetime) activities.

---

* One MET is assumed to be equal to an oxygen uptake of 3.5 milliliters per kilogram of body weight per minute. It is a measure of energy output equal to the resting metabolic rate of an average individual.

Musculoskeletal Conditioning

Musculoskeletal conditioning includes exercises for ensuring that you have an adequate level of flexibility, as well as for developing an appropriate level of muscular fitness. Flexibility was previously discussed in the sections on the warm-up and cool-down phases of an exercise bout. Achieving and maintaining an adequate range of motion should always be an objective of a comprehensive exercise prescription. Flexibility is important for several reasons, including the fact that it reduces an individual's potential for injury and improves an individual's ability to perform certain physical and sports-related tasks.

The warm-up phase of your exercise session should include some type of light warm-up activity to increase both your heart rate and your internal body temperature which is then followed by flexibility exercises which are specifically designed to stretch the musculature around your body's major skeletal joints. Attempting to stretch a cold muscle can be dangerous to the soft tissues surrounding the muscle. No matter how controlled the movement, forcing a muscle through a full normal range of motion (and beyond) without appropriately warming it up is both unsafe and counterproductive.

A general exercise prescription for achieving and maintaining flexibility should adhere to the following guidelines:

- Frequency - daily
- Intensity - to a position of mild discomfort
- Duration - 10-30 seconds for each stretch
- Repetitions - 2-6 for each stretch
- Type - static, with a major emphasis on the low-back and hamstrings area because of the high prevalence of low-back pain syndrome in our society.

Specific guidelines for developing muscular fitness are not nearly as universally accepted as are those for attaining flexibility. Considerable debate exists regarding what constitutes the most appropriate protocol for developing muscular strength and muscular endurance (collectively referred to as muscular fitness). What is generally accepted, however, is the fact that like any system of your body, your muscular system responds to the demands placed upon it. In the exercise arena, the particular form of physical activity that is designed to develop muscular fitness is referred to as resistance training. A growing awareness also exists that resistance training of at least a moderate intensity and sufficient to develop and maintain lean body tissue must be an integral part of a comprehensive (adult) fitness program.

According to the ACSM, one set of 8 to 12 repetitions of 8 to 10 exercises that train the major muscle groups at least two days per week is the recommended minimum amount of resistance training that should be performed to achieve a training effect. Considerable evidence also suggests that in order for your resistance training efforts to be as safe, effective, and efficient as possible, you should:

- Adhere as closely as possible to the specific techniques for performing a particular exercise.
- Exercise to the point of momentary muscular fatigue.
- Perform every exercise through a full range of motion.
- Exercise antagonist muscle groups.
- Perform the eccentric (lowering) portion of a lift in a controlled manner, as well as the concentric (raising phase).
- Include exercises in your training program for all of the major muscle groups of your body—not just a few selected muscle groups.
- Work out (if possible) with a training partner who could, as appropriate, provide you with feedback, support, and motivation.
- Never hold your breath while strength training, since holding your breath can raise your blood pressure to an unsafe level (refer to Valsalva maneuver in Appendix A).

EXERCISING TO AFFECT BODY COMPOSITION

If reducing your level of percent body fat is one of the primary goals of your exercise program, you need to ensure that your exercise program provides a daily caloric expenditure of 300 or more kcal/per session. In addition, you have to watch what you eat. The fundamental determinant of body weight and body composition is caloric balance. Caloric balance entails the difference between caloric intake (energy equivalent of food ingested) and caloric expenditure (energy equivalent of biological work performed). When caloric expenditure exceeds caloric intake, body weight is lost.

Aerobic exercise is the preferred mode of physical activity for fat reduction because it is more efficient than other forms of training (e.g., resistance exercising). The greater efficiency results from the fact that aerobic exercise involves a sustained, high rate of energy expenditure. Keep in mind that the duration and the frequency of exercise are much more important factors than the intensity of exercise for maximizing energy expenditure. As a general rule of thumb, it is suggested that if you want to lose body fat, you should exercise at 50 - 60% of your maximal heart rate reserve, five to seven times per week, for at least 30 minutes per session.

It is encouraging to note that regardless of what form of exercise in which you engage, exercise (at an intensity sufficient to produce a training effect)—all other factors being equal—can physiologically depress your appetite for a short period of time. Individuals who want to consume a diet that will be compatible with their fat-loss goals should adhere to scientifically based dietary recommendations, such as those discussed in chapter 15.

ENVIRONMENTAL CONSIDERATIONS

Environmental factors exist, such as heat, humidity, altitude, and pollution, that can cause HR and perception of effort to increase during an exercise session.

The RPE scale and heart rate are two of the primary indicators that you can use to adjust the intensity and duration of your exercise efforts in diverse environments. In extremely warm conditions, such as very humid and arid climates, the intensity level of your exercise bout should be somewhat restricted. Care should be taken to replace any fluids you lost during and after your exercise sessions. When exercising during extremely cold conditions, you should wear clothing that adequately protects your head (a major avenue of heat loss) and extremities (common sites for frostbite injuries). The intensity and the duration of exercise may also have to be modified (i.e., reduced) when you exercise at high altitudes and in areas with high levels of air pollution (for more information regarding exercise and environmental factors refer to chapter 14).

PROGRAM SUPERVISION

As a basic guideline, apparently healthy, asymptomatic individuals who want to engage in unsupervised exercise programs should have a functional capacity of at least 8 METs. Whatever your fitness level, it is recommended that if you want to engage in an unsupervised exercise program, you should begin with low-intensity exercises, at or below 50% of your functional capacity (60% HR max) and then increase the intensity of your efforts gradually as your body adapts to the stress you've imposed upon it. You should be acutely aware of the signs or symptoms of exertional intolerance (e.g., dizziness, pallor, angina, dypsnea, etc.). It is also in your best interests to have a basic understanding of the fundamental prescription variables of the intensity (THR), duration, and frequency of exercise.

One of the major advantages of joining a health-fitness facility is the fact that they have trained professionals on site to provide you with exercise leadership and guidance. For high-risk or symptomatic individuals, such assistance is extraordinarily valuable. However, these programs are also useful for those individuals who would benefit from hands-on instruction regarding proper exercise technique. In addition, supervised programs can also offer valuable social support for those individuals having difficulty initiating and sustaining lifestyle behavioral changes.

A PRESCRIPTION FOR LIFE

Exercise training can be a valuable tool in improving your relative health and functional status. In order to ensure that you fully receive all of the benefits of a sound exercise program, you need to first identify the existence (if any) of risk factors that may influence the design of your exercise program. Based upon a comprehensive analysis of your personal exercise needs and interests, you should then develop (or have developed for you) an individualized program of exercise that will meet your unique requirements. This program should closely adhere to the primary prescription variables for a sound exercise regimen. Periodically, the manner in which your body has adapted to these variables should be reevaluated. Whenever necessary, you should make adjustments in your personal exercise prescription as appropriate. In so doing, you will be giving yourself a prescription for life . . . a R_x for health and wellness. ❑

BIBLIOGRAPHY •

1. American College of Sports Medicine. *Guidelines for Exercise Testing and Prescription*, 4th Ed. Philadelphia, PA: Lea & Febiger, 1991.
2. American College of Sports Medicine. "Position stand on the recommended quantity and quality of exercise for developing and maintaining cardiorespiratory and muscular fitness in healthy adults." *Med Sci Sports Exerc* 22:264-274, 1990.
3. Astrand, P.O., Rodahl, K. *Textbook of Work Physiology*, 3rd Ed. New York, NY: McGraw-Hill, 1986.
4. Brooks, G.A., Fahey, T.D.. *Exercise Physiology: Human Bioenergetics and Its Applications*. New York, NY: Macmillan Publishing Company, 1985.
5. Franklin, B.A., Gordon, S., Timmis, G.C. (Eds). *Exercise in Modern Medicine*. Baltimore, MD: Williams & Wilkins, 1989.
6. Gledhill, N. "Discussion: Assessment of Fitness." *Exercise, Fitness, and Health: A Consensus of Current Knowledge*. Bouchard, C., et al. (Ed). Champaign, IL: Human Kinetics Publishers, 1990.
7. Heyward. V.H. *Advanced fitness assessment & exercise prescription*, 2nd Ed. Champaign, IL: Human Kinetics Publishers, 1991.
8. Howley, E.T., Franks, B.D.. *Health/Fitness Instructor's Handbook*, 2nd Ed. Champaign, IL: Human Kinetics Publishers, 1992.
9. Nieman, D.C. *Fitness and Sports Medicine: An Introduction*, 2nd Ed. Palo Alto, CA: Bull Publishing Company, 1990.
10. Noble, B.J., Borg, G.A., Jacobs, I., et al. "A category-ratio perceived exertion scale: Relationship to blood and muscle lactate and heart rate." *Med Sci Sports Exerc* 15:523-528, 1983.
11. Painter, P. "Exercise Programming." *Resource Manual for Guidelines for Exercise Testing and Prescription*. American College of Sports Medicine. Philadelphia, PA: Lea & Febiger, 1988.

CHAPTER 12

. . . .

DEVELOPING EXERCISE PRESCRIPTIONS FOR CARDIAC PATIENTS

by

Donald B. Bergey, M.A.
and
Paul M. Ribisl, Ph.D.

• • •

*C*onsiderable research and empirical practice have shown that properly prescribed exercise training can be an effective part of a treatment program for patients with coronary artery disease (CAD). Previous chapters in this book have discussed the benefits and physiological basis of exercise training. The fundamental purpose of exercise training for CAD patients threefold: *primary prevention* (i.e., enhancing positive health), *secondary prevention* (i.e., slowing of the progression of the CAD process) and *rehabilitation* (i.e., restoring normal function). Prescribing exercise for cardiac patients (as well as for other special populations) should follow the basic prescription and training guidelines for healthy populations with the exception of modifications arising from several specific principles which are unique to cardiac patients. This chapter examines the special principles of training which should be applied to CAD patients and offers suggestions regarding how to apply them to an individual training program designed for an individual with CAD.

THE TRAINING STIMULUS

An appropriate discussion of exercise training should initially focus on the size of the training stimulus required to cause a positive physiological adaptation to occur (i.e., an improvement in functional capacity). Most of the literature concerning exercise training suggests specific thresholds which must be exceeded in order to improve functional capacity. The recommended work loads include a range of 40 - 60% of maximal oxygen uptake, 50 - 70% of maximal heart rate response, or the expenditure of 300 kilocalories per exercise session. It is important to realize that the training stimulus for adaptation is based on the *overload principle*. Any work load that is greater (within limits) than that to which any given system is accustomed will produce an increase in the functional capacity of that system. The aforementioned thresholds are actually appropriate work loads for maintenance levels of training in presumably healthy individuals. When training extremely deconditioned diseased individuals, it may be more appropriate to use lower than the standard or "usual" work loads, especially when designing the beginning or "initial" phase of the program.

DEVELOPING A SAFE EXERCISE PRESCRIPTION

Safety is the most important factor that must be addressed when you are developing an exercise prescription for cardiac patients. As you will see in the later discussion, several methods can be used to compute a training work load for CAD patients—each with its advantages and disadvantages. The unyielding guideline for developing an appropriate exercise prescription for an individual with CAD, however, is that the work load must be both safe and realistic for the patient. Making a safe exercise prescription is based on the concept of the level of the "symptom-limited end point." The purpose of a graded exercise (stress) test (GXT) is to evaluate an individual's ability to tolerate gradual increases in the intensity of exercise. The point at which the individual demonstrates an abnormal response pattern to the work load which precludes continuing the exercise is termed the "symptom-limited end point" (i.e., the maximum level of exercise before signs or symptoms of physiological intolerance occur).

Another important part of exercise training is identifying individuals whose participation in exercise programs may be contraindicated (i.e., not recommended) because of specific health/medical conditions they possess. The American College of Sports Medicine (ACSM) in its most recently published guidelines on exercise prescription, developed several criteria which can be used to identify those individuals for whom an exercise program may be contraindicated (refer to Table 12-1).

If you have cardiovascular disease, you should get permission from your physician before you begin an exercise program. Specifically, you should ask your physician if you have any of the contraindicative conditions specified by the ACSM.

Once you begin an exercise program, it is important to know when it is unsafe to continue to exercise. Neil F. Gordon, M.D. and Larry W. Gibbons, M.D., on the staff of the Cooper Clinic in Dallas, Texas, offer the following guidelines[*] concerning what actions you should take if you experience certain symptoms:

---

[*] Authors' Note: These guidelines have been modified from Gordon and Gibbons (1991), p.159.

Table 12-1. Contraindications for Entry into Inpatient and Outpatient Exercise Programs.

The following criteria may be used as contrindications for program entry:

1. Unstable angina (unpredictable or recurring chest pain)
2. Resting systolic blood pressure >200 mm Hg or resting diastolic blood pressure > 100 mm Hg.
3. Orthostatic hypotension (a drop in blood pressure ≥ 20 mm Hg when an individual stands after sitting or lying down)
4. Moderate to severe aortic stenosis (narrowing of the aorta)
5. Acute systemic (whole body) illness or fever
6. Uncontrolled dysrhythmias (abnormal heart rhythms of either the atria or the ventricles)
7. Uncontrolled sinus tachycardia (elevated resting heart rate—greater than 120 bpm)
8. Uncontrolled congestive heart failure
9. Complete (3° A-V) heart block
10. Active pericarditis (inflammation of the membrane covering the heart) or myocarditis (inflammation of the heart muscle)
11. Recent embolism (a traveling blood clot)
12. Thrombophlebitis (inflammation of a vein, often due to a blood clot)
13. Greater than 3 mm resting ST displacement (an ECG abnormality that is indicative of coronary insufficiency)
14. Uncontrolled diabetes
15. Orthopaedic problems that would prohibit exercise

Modified from the American College of Sports Medicine (1991).

- *Pain or discomfort in your chest, abdomen, back, neck, jaw, or arms.* You should never exercise to the point where you develop even a mild form of these symptoms of myocardial ischemia. Even a rating of 1+ ("light, barely noticeable") on the angina scale (refer to Table 12-2) is an indication you've overstepped the bounds of safe exercise. Upon experiencing these symptoms, slow down immediately and notify a rehabilitation staff member. If you're exercising alone and the discomfort doesn't subside within two or three minutes, follow our nitroglycerin guidelines outlined in the following statement. Remember, if ischemia continues for a prolonged period of time, you run the risk of sustaining permanent damage to your heart muscle.
- *If you are alone and you think that it is angina.* Slow down or stop what you are doing immediately. The symptoms should subside within a minute or two, in which case you needn't be unduly alarmed. If your symptoms continue, your physician may have prescribed nitroglycerin tablets (or an oral spray) for just such an occurrence. Take one tablet or dose as directed. If the discomfort is still present after another five minutes, take a second tablet. Again, wait for five minutes. If this doesn't work either, take a final nitroglycerin tablet and call your physician immediately.
- *Unaccustomed shortness of breath during exercise.* For example, if you've always been capable of walking three miles in forty-five minutes with no

breathlessness, then you should be alarmed if suddenly you can't anymore. Notify your doctor.

- *Dizziness or fainting.* During or immediately after exercise, if you get very dizzy and feel as if you are about to faint, it is usually best to lie down flat on your back with your head either level with your body or below your feet.
- *A nauseous sensation during or after exercise.* Treat the same as for dizziness or fainting.
- *An irregular pulse, particularly when it's been regular in past exercise sessions.* If you notice what appear to be either extra heartbeats or missed beats, you may be experiencing premature ventricular contractions (PVC). Once again, summon a staff member or tell your doctor.

Table 12-2. Angina Pain Scale.

1+ Light, barely noticeable
2+ Moderate, bothersome
3+ Severe, very uncomfortable
4+ Most severe pain ever experienced

Everyone who exercises or supervises an exercise program should be familiar with certain warning signs that may indicate that your cardiovascular system is not coping with or adapting to an exercise bout, and that a cardiovascular event may be impending. The ACSM (1991) in its guidelines recently identified specific criteria concerning when an exercise session should be terminated. If any of the following signs or symptoms are experienced, you should stop exercising and seek a medical consultation. Also, no further exercise should be undertaken until you have been seen by a physician. Your exercise session should be terminated if you experience any of the following:

- Excessive Fatigue
- Failure of monitoring equipment
- Light-headedness, confusion, ataxia, pallor, cyanosis, dyspnea, nausea, or any peripheral circulatory insufficiency
- Onset of angina with exercise
- Symptomatic supraventricular tachycardia
- ST displacement (3 mm) horizontal or downsloping from rest
- Ventricular tachycardia (3 or more consecutive PVCs)
- Exercise-induced left bundle branch block
- Onset of second degree and/or third degree A-V block
- R-on-T PVCs (one)
- Frequent multifocal PVCs (30% of the complexes)
- Exercise hypotension (> 20 mm Hg drop in systolic blood pressure during exercise)
- Excessive blood pressure rise: systolic ≥ 220 or diastolic ≥ 110 mm Hg
- Inappropriate bradycardia (drop in heart rate greater than 10 bpm) with increase or no change in work load

Medications are the final consideration concerning how to ensure that your exercise prescription is safe. The safest approach in obtaining an exercise prescription is to consult an experienced or certified exercise physiologist or physician and undergo a GXT. If you are taking any of the class of cardiac medications called beta blockers or calcium channel blockers, you must have a GXT. It is important that you take your medication as you normally would if you are going to use the heart rate method to prescribe the intensity of your exercise program, since these medications alter the heart rate response to exercise. It is best if you can undergo your GXT at about the same time of day as you plan to exercise. The *beta blockers* are Propranolol (Inderal®), Nadolol (Corgard®), Metoprolol (Lopressor®), Atenolol (Tenormin®), Timolol (Blocadren®), Pindolol (Visken®), and Labetalol (Trandate® and Normodyne®). Sectral® and Tenoretic® are combination drugs that also contain a beta-blocker. The *calcium channel blockers* include Nifedipine (Procardia®), Diltiazem (Cardizem®), Verapamil (Calan® and Isoptin®), Bepridil (Vascor®), and Nicardipine HCL (Cardene®).

TYPE OF ACTIVITIES

One of the first decisions to be made concerning an exercise prescription is the type of activity to be used. To make this choice properly, the principle of specificity must be clearly understood. All physical activities can generally be classified into three basic types of exercise: *aerobic, flexibility,* and *resistance. Aerobic* exercise is specific to training the cardiovascular system. It is also the most beneficial type of exercise for making changes in body composition (fat reduction). *Flexibility* exercise is specific for improving the range of motion of the joints and muscles. *Resistance* exercise is specific to training the skeletal muscles for strength and endurance. An overall training program incorporates activities that include each of these types of exercise.

Aerobic exercise is an example of fitness training which involves activities that require your body to be physically moved. No activity is entirely aerobic. The extent to which an activity can be judged as an aerobic exercise depends on how much oxygen is used by the body—a factor which is related to how many of the muscles of the body are used. Fitness activities such as walking/jogging, cycling, swimming, cross country skiing, rowing, stair climbing*, dance, and rope skipping are examples of the most efficient types of aerobic activities because they can be conducted on a non-stop (continuous) basis. They enable you to achieve the most from your training in the least amount of time. Recently conducted research at St. Joseph's Hospital in Phoenix, Arizona, the University of Florida, and Arizona State University indicates that exercising on an independent-step action stair climbing machine may be particularly appropriate for CAD patients because of the fact that it offers weight bearing exercise without the usual accompanying orthopaedic trauma.

---

* Editors' Note: The recently introduced StairMaster® 4000CT™ allows individuals to perform stair climbing exercise within an intensity range of 2.0-8.5 METs.

Most sport activities also involve an aerobic component. A few examples of the more popular athletic endeavors that often place a demand on your aerobic system are basketball, soccer, tennis, racquetball, and even golf (if you walk!). Several dimensions of sport activities diminish their value as aerobic conditioners. First, it is hard to control the intensity level in sports. In most instances, they are usually discontinuous. In addition, if the activities are team sports, you must depend to some degree on other people to get your exercise. Finally, the competitive aspect of sports also makes the intensity level difficult to control.

Flexibility exercise is an example of fitness training which involves activities that move a joint through a full range of movement. The most common type of activity that is used for range of motion is stretching.

Resistance exercise is an example of fitness training which involves activities that require the skeletal muscles to work against a resistance. The most common types of this exercise are weight training and calisthenics.

Most exercise scientists believe that the most important element of your exercise training program is the aerobic component. Accordingly, they conclude that the greatest portion of your workout should be devoted to an aerobic activity. As a general rule, the best aerobic activity is one that you enjoy and will engage in on a regular basis. All factors considered, the best aerobic activity which involves the largest number of people is walking. Range of motion activities involving the major joints in your body should be employed as part of the warm-up that precedes your aerobic activity (but should be applied gently before exercise). On the other hand, range of motion training, which is intended to improve your level of flexibility, should be performed after you engage in aerobic activity (because a warmed muscle can be stretched more safely and effectively). Resistance training should be employed to develop a higher level of muscular fitness, which, in turn, should help alleviate some of the demands on your cardiovascular system that occur with normal, everyday activities.

Training Variables

Several fundamental training variables can be applied to all types of exercise training, including: intensity, duration, frequency, starting level, progression, and warm-up, cool-down. *Intensity* defines how hard the exercise should be performed. Duration defines how long the exercise should be performed. *Frequency* defines how often the exercise should be performed. The *starting level* defines at what training level an exercise program should be initiated. *Progression* defines how to gradually adjust your training program as you become more fit. *Warm-up* and *cool-down* define how to properly prepare the body for exercise and how to enable the body to properly recover from the exercise bout, respectively.

Intensity

The intensity level of the aerobic activity is the most critical part of an exercise prescription for a CAD patient. In order to identify a proper intensity level, a GXT should be administered at approximately the same time of day as the exercise program will be conducted. In the time period immediately after an event (heart attack, open heart surgery, or angioplasty) and before a GXT can be administered, all physical activity can be monitored by using a heart rate upper limit that is equal to the resting heart rate plus 20 beats. This time frame occurs while the individual is still involved in a hospital-based rehab program (Phase I and II or inpatient and outpatient programs). As soon as a GXT is administered, even if it is a "low level" or "discharge" GXT (an exercise stress test which is used only for prognostic purposes), the subsequent exercise level can be set using the GXT results.

The primary focal point in establishing a proper intensity level for the exercise program of a CAD patient involves the concept of the symptom-limited end point. This end point identifies the maximum level of safe exercise that can be performed. This parameter is determined by establishing the level of exercise at which an abnormal response is elicited during the performance of the GXT. If no abnormal responses are seen, then the symptom-limited end point is volitional fatigue—or the highest attainable level of exercise. Once this end point is determined, then the intensity level of the exercise session should be prescribed at a level below this end point. Several methods of prescribing intensity exist—each of which has advantages and disadvantages associated with it. Regardless of which method is used, the concept of the symptom-limited end point is an underlying principle that must be followed.

The simplest method is to use the level of the end point as the maximum level of exercise and allow any training below it. This method has two serious problems, however. By allowing an individual to exercise to the point of an abnormal response, it increases the risk of exceeding this end point, thus entering the "danger zone." Also, by not setting a lower limit, the individual may not be exercising "hard enough" to stimulate a positive training adaptation. A more prudent approach is to adopt a training intensity level that falls within two subjective range limits relative to the end point. This approach enables you to establish a lower limit of training and also to set an upper limit that has a built in "buffer zone" between it and the end point. Three commonly used methods of setting the intensity level based on the symptom-limited end point are:

1. **Oxygen uptake (50-85% of the symptom-limited end point).** The most direct method to set the intensity level is to use the amount of oxygen utilized by the body in an aerobic activity. The measurement most easily used for this method is the MET level. A MET is the metabolic equivalent or amount of oxygen used by your body at rest. Thus, five METs would equal five times the amount of oxygen used at rest. This method is relatively easy to apply. The intensity level is set to equal a range using 50% of the symptom-limited end point as the lower limit of the exercise prescription and 85% of the symptom-limited end point as the upper limit (e.g., an individual with a 10-MET capacity would exercise between 5 and 8.5 METs).

Using METs to establish the intensity level of an exercise program is the most direct method because it uses the rate of oxygen consumption to prescribe the exercise level, which most accurately reflects the intensity of an aerobic activity. Unfortunately, this method has some clear disadvantages that must be understood if it is to be used properly. If the MET level is *estimated* from the work load on the treadmill (or any other ergometer), as opposed to actually *measuring* the work load, the prescription level may be inaccurate because of individual variations in oxygen uptake. (Note: In our laboratory we have found rather large variations in the measured MET levels of our cardiac patients compared to the estimated MET levels.) The major problem with this method is encountered when applying the MET level to a specific bout of exercise. If the aerobic exercise is going to be carried out on an ergometer (treadmill, cycle, arm, or etc.), the MET level becomes very difficult to define. You simply cannot tell someone to walk at six METs, for example. Also, extreme conditions of the environment (heat, cold, and humidity) can change the way the cardiovascular system responds to a given MET level. As a result, the cardiovascular system may be working harder at the same MET level.

2. **Heart rate response (50-85% of symptom-limited end point using the HR-Reserve method).** The heart rate response is an indirect method of applying the exercise prescription, because your heart rate does not accurately reflect the work of your cardiovascular system in all activities. As a result, caution must be taken when using heart rate to determine exercise intensity for non-aerobic activities or activities that do not have a large aerobic component. When heart rate is used with aerobic activities, however, it is probably the best method, because it is the easiest to apply and will reflect the effect of the environment on the cardiovascular system more accurately. Two methods are commonly used for computing training heart rate: the percent of heart rate-maximum (% HR-max), and the heart rate reserve method (HR-Reserve). The HR-Reserve method is also known as the Karvonen method. The % HR-max method is applied by simply computing a given percent of a set heart rate-maximum (e.g., the symptom-limited end point). The HR-Reserve method uses the following formula:

$$THR = [(SLHR - RHR) \times (CI/100)] + RHR$$
where:
    THR = Training heart rate
    SLHR = Symptom limited end point heart rate
    RHR = Resting heart rate
    CI = Conditioning intensity

The HR-Reserve method has two features which make it particularly appropriate for use with cardiac patients:

- Heart rates computed by this formula very closely approximate heart rates computed by using the relationship to oxygen uptake.
- If the resting heart rate is not used to compute the training heart rate, it is possible that the training heart rate will be actually lower than the resting heart rate for some patients.

3. **The Borg Scale or RPE (Rating of Perceived Exertion) (11-14 on the 15-point scale or 3-5 on the 10-point scale).** The RPE scales developed by Swedish psychologist, Gunnar Borg, enable individuals to monitor the intensity level of an exercise bout by rating how hard they perceive themselves to be exercising (refer to Table 11-1).

Caution should be used if applying RPE levels with patients just beginning an exercise program, especially if the individuals have not engaged in exercise training for a significant period of time. The RPE scale is appropriate for use after patients have exercised for some time and if they change the dosage of a beta blocker or calcium channel blocker medication. While the change in dosage will affect their heart rate response, it will not affect their interpretation of the RPE scale.

Both the Heart Rate Reserve and the RPE scale should be explained to the patient (refer to Figure 12-1). Patients can be safely monitored in an outpatient program through either self monitoring of their heart rate or through the use of a HR monitoring technique which employs a tool specifically designed to measure HR (refer to Figure 12-2).

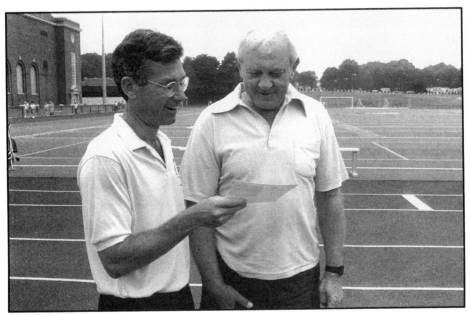

Figure 12-1.   Instructing the patient in what constitutes a safe level of exercise using the heart rate reserve method.

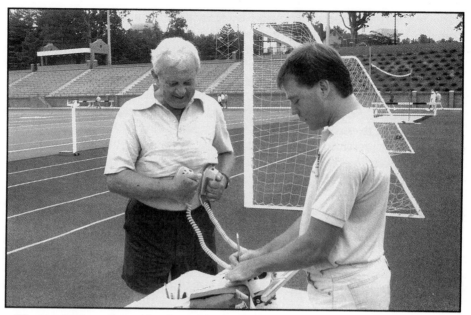

Figure 12-2. Spot checking the heart rate of a patient using (Physio Control Lifepak) paddles.

DURATION (30 ≥ MINUTES/DAY)

The duration of an activity, which should be at least 30 minutes, applies directly to the stimulus phase of the program and is exclusive of the time spent in warm-up and cool-down. This time period can be used intermittently (especially by extremely deconditioned individuals, or those just beginning an exercise program) or split up among two or three sessions in a single day.

Duration is best quantified in terms of time, as opposed to distance. The only appropriate method for equating training routines using different activities is to compare intensity as a work rate and duration as time. Distance will not equate among different activities. Jogging three miles, for example, does not compare with swimming three miles or cycling three miles. Training at a given heart rate for a given period of time will produce approximately the same cardiovascular training stimulus, even if you're performing a different type of aerobic activity.

FREQUENCY (3 OR 4 DAYS/WEEK)

The frequency of training defines how many times or days per week that a given work bout should be performed. An important principle of frequency that should be understood involves the necessity for alternating easy and hard training days/sessions. This guideline suggests that an individual should not engage in "hard" training sessions for two or more consecutive days. A hard training session may be defined as one involving either high intensity or long duration. It should also be understood that "easy" and "hard" are relative terms and must be judged according to the individual. An "easy" day for a *beginning* or *low functional capacity* patient might be considered to be a day of light or no exercise, or if weight bearing exercise is the usual training, a session using a non-weight bearing exercise.

While research has found that two days per week of exercise training are required to *maintain* functional capacity, three days and possibly four days of training per week are probably needed to *improve* functional capacity. Depending on whether your exercise program is designed for maintenance or improvement, the aforementioned are the *optimal* training frequencies. Five to seven days per week can be used by patients if they are engaging in very low intensity and very low duration sessions, or by patients who have very high functional capacity and have been training for a long period of time. In the latter case, caution must be observed because of the high incidence of orthopaedic injuries that often occurs in individuals who exercise on a high frequency basis.

STARTING LEVEL (1 - 6 WEEKS)

Setting the initial work bout in an exercise program is a very important part of the exercise prescription. If the first training session that a patient performs is too difficult, the experience can be very discouraging and even dangerous. If the first session is too easy, the patient might not perceive any benefit from the program. As a result, establishing a work load that is between these two extremes is the ideal approach. Because setting a work load is always an "educated guess," it is better to err on the side of conservatism. As a basic rule of thumb, it is better to establish an exercise level that will allow a patient to succeed, rather than fail. This is where the "art" of exercise prescription comes in. The starting level should last from one to six weeks. How to set the initial level and how long it should last depends on a number of factors, including: age, exercise history, body weight, and the functional capacity of the patient. The basic rule is that the older, the less active, the heavier, and the more unfit the individual, the lower the starting level. Probably the most important fact to know about patients is how much exercise they have been doing before starting in your program. This information enables you to set an exercise level that is consistent with what the patient has already been doing. The following discussion relates how the training principles can be manipulated to set a proper starting level.

- *Type of Activity.* Consider using weight bearing activities with beginning patients, especially if the patient is a larger than normal individual (large because of fat tissue or muscle tissue). Weight bearing activities (e.g., running, walking) generally cause more stress on the joints and muscles than non-weight bearing activities.[*]

- *Intensity.* Do not be afraid of using lower than the normal or traditional levels of intensity (50%) to start an exercise program for a patient. Remem-

---

[*] Editors' Note: The StairMaster® 4000PT® and the StairMaster® 4000CT® offer a means for providing weight-bearing exercise with little or no orthopaedic stress.

ber that the training stimulus depends on the overload principle, and a 20% intensity may represent an overload for some patients.

• *Duration.* Consider using intermittent programs of walking/rest for beginning patients. It your client has the flexibility to exercise at different times of the day, another good plan is to split up work bouts into two or three sessions a day. For example, a 30-minute work bout can be split into a 15-minute session in the morning and a 15-minute session in the afternoon. Or a 30-minute work bout can be split into a 10-minute session in the morning, a 10-minute session at noon, and a 10-minute session in the late afternoon.

• *Frequency.* Remember the principle of alternating easy and hard training days. (Note: An easy day for a beginner may mean a day off.)

SLOW PROGRESSION (UP TO 6 MONTHS)

A sensible progression of the exercise prescription should be controlled by the training levels that move a patient from the starting level to the maintenance level. A safe rate of progression incorporates small increases in work loads that are adopted in a time schedule that enables positive physiological adaptations to take place. The period of time necessary to develop desirable baseline (starting) levels of fitness can take up to six months, depending on the goals of the individual. How fast a patient progresses should generally adhere to the same guidelines for setting the starting level, with the critical issue being how long to spend at each level. The general rule is that your body takes two weeks of training to adapt to a new work load. An example of a walking progression for a cardiac patient is presented in Table 12-3. The number of sessions required at each level can be adjusted both initially and throughout the training regimen according to the health/fitness status of, and the relative rate of adaptation by, the patient.

Table 12-3. Sample Walking Progression Program.

NAME_____ DATE STARTED _____

# of Sessions	Walking Routine	Dates
_____	Walk 5 min./Rest 3-5 min. (Repeat x 2)	_____
_____	Walk 5 min./Rest 3-5 min. (Repeat x 3)	_____
_____	Walk 5 min./Rest 3-5 min. (Repeat x 4)	_____
_____	Walk 10 min./Rest 3-5 min. (Repeat x 2)	_____
_____	Walk 10 min./Rest 3-5 min. (Repeat x 3)	_____
_____	Walk 15 min./Rest 3-5 min. (Repeat x 2)	_____
_____	Walk 20 min./Rest 3-5 min./Walk 15 min.	_____
_____	Walk 25 min./Rest 3-5 min./Walk 10 min.	_____
_____	Walk 30 min./Rest 3-5 min./Walk 5 min.	_____
_____	Walk 35 min./Rest 3-5 min.	_____
_____	Walk 40 min. (Maintenance)	_____

WARM-UP (10 - 15 MINUTES)

The work bout or stimulus phase should be preceded by an adequate *warm-up* session. The purpose of the warm-up is to ensure that the cardiovascular system is prepared to function safely at an elevated level and that the joints and muscles are prepared for the exercise bout without undue risk of injury. Accordingly, a warm-up session should consist of two parts.

The first part of the warm-up period should raise your body core temperature. The best way to accomplish this is with the same activity that is going to be used in the stimulus phase, but performed at a lower level of intensity. Research has shown that even normal, healthy cardiovascular systems can demonstrate ischemic responses in reaction to abrupt and extreme increases in exercise intensity. This issue becomes an even more important safety factor when training cardiac patients. This part should last from five to ten minutes. The second part of the warm-up phase should include some very gentle range of motion activities such as light, static stretching. Your body temperature needs to be elevated in order to allow for safer and more productive stretching. The older the individual is and the earlier in the day the activities are being performed, the more time should be devoted to the warm-up and stretching.

COOL-DOWN (10 - 25 MINUTES)

A *cool-down* session should follow the *stimulus* phase of the exercise bout. A cool-down phase should consist of the same two parts as the warm-up period. Similar to the warm-up, the first part of a cool-down should involve approximately five to ten minutes of the same aerobic activity performed at a lower level of intensity. This approach to cooling down is designed to permit your cardiovascular system to return to its resting functional status without compromising adequate circulation to your vital organs (heart and brain). The second part of a cool-down session involves performing additional repetitions of range of motion activities. Such exercise has several potential benefits. For example, some evidence exists to support the contention that post-activity stretching decreases the muscle soreness that is common in individuals who are starting an exercise program. Furthermore, because the muscles and joints are sufficiently warmed, it is also an ideal time to utilize a more vigorous stretching routine in order to train for increasing flexibility.

RESISTANCE TRAINING

The activities of everyday life require that you perform resistance exercises. For example, whenever you move your body or an object through space, you are doing a resistance exercise. Traditionally, heavy resistance exercise was perceived by members of the exercise science and medical communities to be more of a "strain" than a training stimulus on the cardiovascular system. As a result, for a number of years, resistance work was seldom prescribed for cardiac patients. In recent years, however, sufficient research has demonstrated conclusively that training the skeletal muscles to perform resistance exercise can, in fact, reduce the "strain" on the cardiovascular system.

The American College of Sports Medicine has adopted a position in support of the value of sound resistance training for CAD patients. The ACSM (1991) guidelines suggest that the following exclusion criteria for resistance training be used to identify individuals for whom resistance training would not be appropriate:
- Abnormal hemodynamic responses or ischemic changes on the electrocardiogram during graded exercise.
- Poor left ventricular function.
- Peak exercise capacity < 6 METs.
- Uncontrolled hypertension or dysrhythmias.

Resistance training to develop muscular fitness should adhere to the same basic training principles as for cardiovascular fitness. The application of these principles to resistance activities is different, however, than for aerobic activities.

Intensity. The intensity of a resistance activity is measured by the resistance against which the muscle must move. Heavy resistances ($\geq$ 60% of the maximum amount of weight that can be lifted one time) should be avoided by cardiac patients.

Duration. The duration of a resistance activity is measured by the number of times that the object is lifted. This number is referred to as the repetitions (REPs) performed. As with aerobic activity, there is an inverse relationship between intensity (weight) and duration (repetitions). The traditional DeLorme theory of resistance training theorizes that the higher the weight and the lower the repetitions, the more the training will increase muscular strength. By the same token, the lower the weight and the higher the repetitions, the more the training will increase muscular endurance.* The most commonly followed guideline for cardiac patients is to perform 10 to 15 REPs. Two or three sets (i.e., groups of repetitions of an exercise movement performed consecutively, without rest, until a given number, or momentary exhaustion, is reached) of each routine are also normally recommended.

Frequency. If more intense strength training (using heavier weights) is being performed, then the training should be done only every second or third day. At lower levels of relative resistance, the issue of adequate time to recover is not as critical.

Starting level. A critical element in developing a safe, sensible resistance training program for cardiac patients involves determining what initial level of resistance should be used for each exercise. Initial weights should not be more

---

* Editors' Note: The ACSM (1991) recommends that an effective protocol for developing either muscular strength or muscular endurance is to perform a single set of 8-12 repetitions of each exercise.

than 40 to 50% of the one-repetition maximal level (1-RM) of a patient. While 1-RM *testing* has been shown to be a relatively safe technique for most CAD patients, a more useful and prudent way is the "Titration" method. This method involves having patients start with 10 REPs with a lighter more comfortable weight, and then progressing to 15 REPs each training session. At their next workout, they raise the resistance level for a specific exercise to the next highest weight for 10 REPs of an initial set. During the session, they again progress to being able to perform one set of 15 REPs. This process continues until the patient identifies the level of resistance that is appropriate to the individual's training objectives.

Slow progression. The individual can progress to the next highest level of resistance for a particular exercise when 15 REPs of a weight can be performed for two or three sets without significant strain. The initial number of repetitions that should be performed at the new level of resistance is usually ten. If the individual can't perform at least ten, the amount of increase was too high or undertaken too soon.

Safety is the most crucial issue attendant to resistance training for cardiac patients. Specific guidelines for the safe and effective application of resistance training for cardiac patients have been developed by the American Association of Cardiovascular and Pulmonary Rehabilitation (1991), including the following:

- To prevent soreness and injury, initially choose a weight that will allow an individual to comfortably perform 10 to 12 REPs of an exercise. In general, this level of resistance will correspond to a level which is approximately 40 to 60 percent of the maximum weight load that can be lifted in one REP. High-risk adults and low-risk cardiac patients should select an initial weight load that can be lifted for 12 to 15 REPs.
- Generally, two to three sets of each exercise are recommended.
- Don't strain! Ratings of perceived exertion (6-20 scale) should not exceed "fairly light" (11) to "somewhat hard" (13) during lifting.
- Avoid breath holding. Breathe normally at all times.
- Increase the amount of resistance lifted by 2.5 to 10 pounds when 10 to 12 repetitions can be comfortably accomplished; for high-risk adults and cardiacs, the weight should be increased only after the individual can easily manage 12 to 15 repetitions of an exercise.
- Raise the weight to a count of two, and lower the weight gradually to a count of four; emphasize complete extension of the limbs when lifting.
- Include exercises for all of the major muscle groups of the body.
- Organize the resistance training program so that muscles are generally exercised in a largest-to-smallest order two to three times per week.
- Avoid excessive hand gripping when possible, since this may evoke an excessive blood pressure response to lifting.
- Stop exercising in the event of any contraindicative warning signs or symptoms, especially dizziness, abnormal heart rhythm, unusual shortness of breath, and/or chest pain.
- Don't rest for an extended period of time between either the exercises or the sets of exercises.

• Whenever possible, all patients should be monitored and their responses recorded (heart rate, symptoms, etc.) to the resistance exercise following each set. ❑

BIBLIOGRAPHY •

1. American Association of Cardiovascular and Pulmonary Rehabilitation. *Guidelines for Cardiac Rehabilitation Programs.* Champaign, IL: Human Kinetics Publishers, 1991.
2. American College of Sports Medicine. *Guidelines For Exercise Testing and Prescription,* 4th Ed. Philadelphia, PA: Lea & Febiger, 1991.
3. Brannon, F.J., Geyer, M.J., Foley, M.W. *Cardiac Rehabilitation.* Philadelphia, PA: F. A. Davis Company, 1988.
4. Fardy, P.S., Yanowitz, F.G., Wilson, P.K. *Cardiac Rehabilitation, Adult Fitness, and Exercise Testing,* 2nd Ed. Philadelphia, PA: Lea & Febiger, 1988.
5. Gordon, N.F., Gibbons, L.W. *The Cooper Clinic Cardiac Rehabilitation Program.* New York, NY: Simon and Schuster, 1990.
6. Hall, L.K., Meyer, G.C. (Eds). *Cardiac Rehabilitation: Exercise testing and prescription,* Vol. II. Champaign, IL: Human Kinetics Publishers, 1988.
7. Hall, L.K., Meyer, G.C., Hellerstein, H.K. (Eds). *Cardiac Rehabilitation: Exercise testing and prescription.* Champaign, IL: Human Kinetics Publishers, 1984.
8. McKelvie, R.S., McCartney, N. "Weightlifting training in cardiac patients: Considerations." *Sports Med* 10(6):355-364, 1990.
9. Wilson, P. K. "Cardiac rehabilitation: Then and now." *Phys Sportsmed* 16(9):75-84, 1988.

CHAPTER 13

DEVELOPING EXERCISE PRESCRIPTIONS FOR OLDER ADULTS

by

M. Elaine Cress, Ph.D.
and
Dennis Colacino, Ph.D.

• • •

*T*he ranks of the elderly are rapidly increasing. There are currently 30 million Americans over the age of 65 (12% of the population). If current trends continue, the elderly are projected to represent 20% of the population by the year 2030. Inescapably, as individuals become older, they experience a decline in the function of most physiologic systems of the body. These normal, yet irreversible, physiologic changes which occur over an individual's lifetime are collectively referred to as the aging process.

EFFECTS OF TIME

The cardiovascular system undergoes several changes as a person ages. These changes, coupled with alterations occurring in both the pulmonary and muscular systems, are responsible for a steady decline in maximal oxygen uptake ($\dot{V}O_2$ max) as a person ages (refer to Figure 13-1). Some of the more prominent changes which occur include:

- A decrease in cardiac muscle size and heart volume, which decreases the heart's ability to pump blood.
- A decrease in the sympathetic nerve activity to the heart which results in a lower attainable maximal heart rate and a reduced strength of heart contraction.
- A decrease in the elasticity of the major blood vessels which results in elevated blood pressure (at rest and during activity).

Figure 13-1. Aging is accompanied by a decrease in cardiorespiratory and musculosketetal function. Many of these changes also occur during the transition from a trained to an untrained state. *Modified from Nieman, D.C. (1990).*

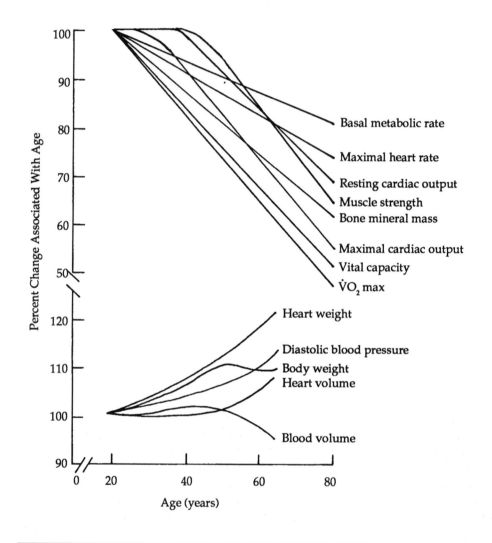

Aging also produces some major changes in the pulmonary system. A decline in the structural integrity of the alveoli (the functional unit of the lung) reduces the surface area for gas exchange and thereby limits the diffusion capacity for oxygen to the blood. The elasticity of lung tissue and the strength of respiratory muscles decrease and rib cage stiffness increase with aging. The combined effect is an increase in the energy cost of breathing.

The musculoskeletal system undergoes numerous changes as individuals age. A progressive, steady decline in muscle mass and strength (especially of the lower extremities) occurs with age, leading to deficiencies in gait and balance, loss of functional mobility, increased risk of falling and ultimately a loss of independence. Muscle mitochondrial and enzymatic changes, which reduce muscle respiratory capacity (the muscle's ability to extract oxygen from the blood), occur as a result of aging. Aging is associated with a decrease in bone mineral content and mass (this occurs in both sexes), increasing the older person's risk for osteoporosis and bone fractures. With age, increased stiffness of connective tissue results in a loss of joint flexibility and mobility.

The aforementioned is but a brief overview of some of the various physiologic changes that occur with aging. While the fact that most bodily systems experience some form of decline in functioning presents a somewhat dismal picture, there is good news. A significant portion (some estimates have been as high as 50%) of the physiologic decline typically seen with aging can be attributed to disuse atrophy resulting from physical inactivity. In the words of Hippocrates, the father of medicine, "All parts of the body which have function, if used in moderation and exercised in labors in which each is accustomed, become thereby healthy, well developed, and age more slowly; but if unused and left idle, they become liable to disease, defective in growth, and age quickly."

EFFECTS OF EXERCISE

A critical question concerning the aging process involves whether exercise can slow down the biological changes that occur over the course of an individual's lifetime. The answer appears to be a resounding "yes," although the extent to which exercising on a regular basis can affect the response of certain bodily systems to aging is generally unknown. At the least, a physically active lifestyle can positively affect age-associated declines that in large part may be attributed to the fact that most people become less active as they age.

CARDIORESPIRATORY ADAPTATIONS

Numerous investigative efforts have shown that elderly individuals who exercise can achieve a demonstrable cardiorespiratory training effect. For example, even though $\dot{V}O_2$ max declines in everyone as we get older, physically active individuals are able to slow their average rate of decline in $\dot{V}O_2$ max to a level approximately half that of their sedentary counterparts. This means that an active 65-year-old person can be as aerobically fit as a 45-year-old sedentary person. In addition, older individuals who remain physically active do not experience the typical rise in blood pressure that occurs with aging.

MUSCULOSKELETAL ADAPTATIONS

Several recent studies support the belief that strength training can forestall the rate of deterioration of the musculoskeletal system in older persons. In these studies, individuals who engaged in a resistance training program maintained their strength. In fact, strength levels actually increased dramatically. In comparison, inactive individuals typically show a 20 percent loss in strength by age 65. Participants in the experimental training in these studies also incurred an increase in muscle mass, in contrast to the decrease in their inactive counterparts that traditionally occurs. Finally, proper strength training has been documented to maintain or increase joint flexibility, since it involves having an individual exercise through a full range of motion.

BODY COMPOSITION ADAPTATIONS

Exercise can reduce the accumulation of body fat that accompanies aging and can slow, if not reverse, the substantial loss of fat-free mass that usually goes hand-in-hand with the increase in body fat. Older people can maintain the level of body fat they had in their youth if they remain consistently physically active and maintain an appropriate diet throughout their lives. Researchers suggest that proper strength training can attenuate the loss of lean muscle mass levels that often accompanies aging.

LIFESTYLE CHANGES

Exercise on a regular basis can have a positive effect on the overall quality of life in older adults in many ways, including:

- Regular exercise can provide older individuals with the functional capacity (attendant to having minimal levels of fitness in each of the primary components of physical fitness) necessary to perform basic living tasks, such as shopping, ambulation, personal care, and cooking meals.
- Physical activity can help an older person adapt to the changing social roles that sometimes accompany advancing age. For example, an activity program may replace work in the life of the individual.
- Social interaction can be promoted through exercise programs. Physical activity can help in adjusting to a traumatic event—e.g., retirement, the death of a loved one—by providing an avenue for social interaction and combating feelings of depression.
- Regular exercise can assist individuals in adjusting to retirement. Exercise, for example, can provide a relatively inexpensive activity for those on a reduced income. In addition, maintaining physical fitness enables older persons to remain independent, thereby incurring fewer of the costs for assistance that arise if they need home management and personal care.
- Old age frequently requires that older people must scale down their housing or move into an apartment or retirement community. Since many retirement communities do not take people who are physically dependent, maintaining physical fitness enables individuals to have more diverse options in their possible physical living arrangements. In several multi-level retirement communities, for example, the average cost for assisted living (e.g., help in making the bed, meals, home finances) is estimated to be more than double the monthly average cost required to live independently.

Developing An Exercise Program

The first step is to ensure that the individual is medically safe to exercise. This involves seeing a physician and undergoing a physical examination and evaluation <u>before</u> an exercise program is initiated. The extent of the evaluation depends on the individual's age and health status. Men over age 40, women over age 50, and all individuals at high risk (e.g., having one or more of the following risk factors—smoking, hypertension, high blood cholesterol, obesity, stress, family history of medical problems, diabetes) are strongly encouraged to undergo a physician-supervised, graded exercise test.

The next step is to develop a sound exercise program based on scientifically documented information. A sound exercise prescription enables an individual to achieve as much as possible (effectiveness), as quickly as possible (efficiency), and most importantly, without undue risk of injury. If an exercise regimen is to be relatively risk-free for older individuals, it must be tailored to their age, gender, and current level of fitness.

A safety-oriented exercise program also involves starting at a level of intensity appropriate for the individual and then progressing gradually. The temptation to do too much too soon should be avoided. Moderation is essential. A major cause of musculoskeletal injuries is overuse—placing demands on the individual's body that the body simply is not capable of handling. A sound exercise program always includes provisions for stretching the major joints of the body before and after exercising. It also ensures that the individual get proper rest along with exercise. Rest enables individuals to recover from the demands of exercise placed on their bodies.

The final step is for individuals to listen to their bodies. They must respond accordingly to specific warning signals of exertional intolerance. These warning signs are grouped into three general categories according to their severity.

Category I: If individuals experience any of the following symptoms, they should stop exercising immediately and consult a physician before resuming exercise:

- Abnormal heart rhythm (irregular pulse; fluttering, pumping or palpitations in the chest or throat; a sudden burst of rapid heart beats or a very sudden slowing of the pulse).
- Pain or pressure in the arm or throat or in the middle of the chest (either during or after exercising).
- Acute heat or overuse-related signals (dizziness; light-headedness; sudden loss of coordination; mental disorientation; profuse sweating; glassy stare; unnatural pallor; blueness; fainting).

Category II: If an individual experiences any of the following symptoms and the suggested (listed) remedy doesn't work for the individual, the person should see a physician before exercising again:

- Persistent rapid heart rate (remedy—keep the heart rate at the lower end of the individual's aerobic training zone for several minutes at the start of the exercise session and then increase it very slowly as the individual continues to exercise).
- Flare-up of musculosketetal conditions, such as osteoarthritis (remedy—stop exercising until the condition subsides; individuals should take their normal medicine for their condition).

Category III: The following warning signs can usually be handled without consulting a physician:

- Vomiting or nausea after exercising (remedy—reduce the intensity level of the present and future exercise bouts; take a more gradual cooling-down period after exercising).
- Extreme breathlessness that lasts more than ten minutes after the individual has stopped exercising (remedy—individuals should never exercise to the point where they're too breathless to talk while they're exercising).
- Prolonged fatigue or insomnia (remedy—exercise at the lower end of the aerobic training zone for the next several exercise bouts, and then begin to gradually increase the exercise intensity level).
- Side-stitch (remedy—sit, lean forward, and attempt to push the abdominal organs against the diaphragm).

Prescribing Aerobic Exercise

The general principles of exercise prescription (refer to chapter 11) apply to individuals of all ages. However, the wide range of health and fitness levels observed among older adults make prescribing exercise for them more difficult. Great care must be taken in establishing the type, intensity, duration, and frequency of exercise.

Type

Selecting a mode of exercise for developing aerobic fitness can involve several factors. For most older persons (particularly those who have been sedentary), the exercise modality should be one that does not impose significant orthopaedic stress on the aged musculoskeletal system. Research has also shown that the activity should be something that is accessible, convenient, and enjoyable to the participant—all factors directly related to exercise adherence. Among the more popular methods of exercising that older adults use to develop aerobic fitness are the following:

Walking. Walking is an excellent form of exercise for young and old alike. It is beneficial for older adults for several reasons: it doesn't require learning a new skill; it can be done almost anywhere, indoors or outdoors; it doesn't require special clothing or equipment, except for a good pair of walking shoes; and, finally, if performed on a treadmill, it can be an activity in which preselected physiological and performance measures can be monitored by the person or an exercise specialist. The primary disadvantage of walking is the fact that a certain amount of orthopaedic stress is imposed on the skeletal joints of the user.

Stair Climbing. Recently, researchers at the University of Florida have shown that not only do older adults incur substantial improvement in both cardiorespiratory endurance and lower extremity musculoskeletal fitness as a result of exercising on independent step-action stair climbing machines, they also appear to greatly enjoy this form of exercise. Unlike the traditional forms of weight-bearing activities (e.g., walking, running, exercising on a treadmill), considerable evidence suggests that exercising on an independent step-action stair climbing machine does not impose injurious orthopaedic stress on the joints. Given the fact that lower-body musculoskeletal fitness is critical to the maintenance of functional mobility in the elderly, an orthopaedically safe weight-bearing exercise modality, such as an independent step-action stair climbing machine, can offer invaluable benefits to the exerciser. The primary downside of stair climbing is that an orthopaedically safe independent step-action stair climbing machine is relatively expensive.

Water Exercise. Swimming and water aerobic exercise (aquatic) classes offer certain advantages for older adults. The benefit most frequently cited is the fact that water-based activities have lower musculoskeletal injury rates and greater joint range of motion than most traditional weight-bearing activities. In addition, exercising in water offers the opportunity to engage in both upper and lower body muscular resistance exercise. The most obvious downside of water-based activities involves the need for access to a pool and the fact that an individual may not feel comfortable around water. Also, aquatic exercise classes do not promote positive bone adaptations since water-based activities are not weight bearing.

Stationary Cycling. Stationary cycling is a particularly safe modality for older adults. The weather is not a factor indoors. No substantial concern exists concerning the possibility of an older adult falling off the cycle. If adapting to the seat is a problem, equipping the cycle with an extra large seat tends to minimize the discomfort for people unaccustomed to a bicycle seat. If excessive fatigue in the user's thigh muscles is a problem (given the role of the quadriceps in exercise cycling), gradually increasing the exercise duration while reducing or holding intensity (i.e., pedal resistance) constant may minimize the problem of using a stationary cycle that employs wind resistance (e.g., the Windracer® exercise cycle). Stationary cycling has at least two significant shortcomings. First, an exercise cycle is needed. A quality exercise cycle can either be purchased or be part of the equipment offering of a health-fitness facility. Either option may be relatively expensive. Second, and more importantly, as a non-weight bearing activity, exercise cycling does not offer the beneficial effects on bone mass that weight-bearing activity does. The aerobic portion of the cycling exercise session may be broken into 10-minute segments and interspersed with 10-minute bouts of other forms of aerobic exercise, such as walking, simulated stair climbing, etc.

Aerobic Dance. Aerobic dance has several significant advantages and disadvantages for the older population. A list of the advantages includes: aerobic dance sessions are structured, yet social, events; aerobic dance can improve body awareness and can approximate everyday motions such as bending and reaching; aerobic dance exercise provides an opportunity to work on posture, gait and balance; and, finally, aerobic dance enables exercises involving coordination and flexibility to be integrated effectively with aerobic fitness activities. Among the more important possible disadvantages of this form of exercise are the following: an aerobic dance class must be comprised of persons with similar capabilities (to ensure safety); the risk of acute or chronic injuries is high; and the fitness benefits from class to class are not as predictable as from more structured forms of aerobic exercise (e.g., cycling, stair climbing, etc.) Finally, aerobic dance is more dependent than other forms of aerobic exercise on the skills of the exercise leader for direction, safety, motivation, and ultimate effectiveness.

INTENSITY

Perhaps the most important and, at the same time, potentially the most problematic training variable is exercise intensity. Exercise intensity must be sufficient to stress (overload) the cardiovascular, pulmonary, and musculoskeletal systems without overtasking them. In general, the intensity of exercise coincides with the training heart rate. Training heart rate (THR) is often determined by taking a straight percentage of age-predicted maximal heart rate (i.e., 220 minus age). This method of defining exercise intensity can, however, be very misleading in older individuals. High variability exists for maximal heart rates in persons over 55 years of age (maximal heart rates can range from as low as 100 bpm to as high as 190 bpm). Training heart rates calculated on the basis of age-predicted maximal heart rates can either underestimate or overestimate the exercise intensity. Thus, it is always better to use an accurate measurement of maximal heart rate (MHR) rather than age-predicted MHR.

The heart rate reserve method (Karvonen) is recommended for establishing THR in older individuals. Since MHR decreases and resting heart rate (RHR) increases with age, it would be possible to compute a THR that is lower than RHR, if the RHR is not used in the computation of the THR. The Karvonen method calculates the THR by using a percentage of the heart rate reserve as presented in chapter 11, (the difference between the maximum and resting heart rates).

The recommended level of exercise intensity for an older adult is 50-70% of maximal heart rate reserve (this also closely approximates a similar percentage of maximal oxygen uptake). Since many older persons suffer from a variety of medical conditions, a conservative approach to prescribing aerobic exercise is usually warranted. Individuals with a relatively low level of functional capacity should initially engage in aerobic exercise at an intensity range of 50-60% of maximal HRR, which can then be very gradually increased over a period of two to three months. For individuals with a normal level of functional capacity, an intensity range of 60-70 of maximal HRR is appropriate. When setting exercise intensity for older individuals, the general rule is "start low and go slow."

DURATION

Exercise duration and intensity go hand in hand. An increase in one often requires a decrease in the other. The prescription for duration is usually expressed in terms of time, distance, or calories. All three are interrelated. Most people prefer, however, to use time as their indicator of duration because of its comparative simplicity of use. Other than a watch or access to a clock, nothing is required except the ability to tell time.

The ACSM guideline (aimed at primarily healthy younger to middle-age adults) for duration recommends that an aerobic exercise workout take between 20 and 60 minutes. The goal of most older adults should be 20 to 30 minutes of sustained activity. Less than 20 minutes is often sufficient to provide for a significant training effect for many sedentary older people. During the initial stages of an exercise program, some older adults may have difficulty sustaining aerobic exercise for more than 10 minutes. For such individuals one viable option may be to perform the exercise in several 10-minute bouts throughout the day. If the exercise session is segmented, the individual should be encouraged to perform it at regularly scheduled times, so as to enhance compliance and adherence. For individuals with a low functional capacity (2-3 METs*), it may actually be preferable to schedule frequent 10-minute bouts of exercise throughout the day. Older persons who have a capacity of 3-5 METs may benefit from an exercise prescription involving two, ten-minute (at the minimum) bouts of aerobic sessions. To avoid injury and ensure safety, older individuals should raise the difficulty level of their workouts primarily through increases in exercise duration.

FREQUENCY

Researchers have found that an individual needs to exercise aerobically 3-5 days a week in order to achieve the intended training effect. Exercising less than twice a week has been found to produce little or no meaningful training response. By the same token, exercising more than five days a week results in little or no further improvement in an individual's maximum oxygen uptake level. In fact, the amount of positive change in a person's aerobic fitness level begins to plateau when the individual exercises more than three to four days per week. During the initial stages of weight-bearing aerobic exercise, exercising on alternate days is recommended to gradually give the individual's body an opportunity to adapt to the stresses being imposed upon it (thereby reducing the likelihood of an "overuse" injury). For persons who want to exercise aerobically on a daily basis, alternating between weight bearing (e.g., walking or stair climbing) and non-weight bearing (e.g., exercise cycling) is advised.

---

*One MET is assumed to be equal to an oxygen uptake of 3.5 millimeters per kilogram of body weight per minute. It is a measure of energy output equal to the resting metabolic rate of an average individual.

PRESCRIBING RESISTANCE TRAINING

The effects of resistance training and various strength training protocols have been relatively well-defined for younger populations. Recently published research findings suggest that muscular fitness (muscular strength and muscular endurance) offers considerable benefits to older adults. For example, it appears that strength training may enable elderly individuals (particularly women) to be able to perform their daily living tasks with greater ease, as well as leading to a heightened sense of self-confidence and self-worth. A certain level of muscular fitness is critical for individuals to retain their independence. Individuals obviously want and need to perform certain daily tasks for themselves. It is believed that strength training provides significant skeletal benefits for men and women of all ages. While the thought of "pumping up" to older adults might seem somewhat strange, it appears to be an inescapable fact that an appropriate level of muscular fitness is integral to ensuring that individuals are able to spend their latter years in a self-functioning, dignified manner.

Although the ability of older adults to realize significant strength gains has been documented, the specifics of resistance training protocols for older adults have not been adequately addressed. For example, considerable research has shown that achieving a training effect for muscular fitness does not have to involve extended periods of time in the weight room, lifting massive amounts of free weights. On the contrary, calisthenics using body weight to stimulate an overload of the muscle, weighted and non-weighted stair climbing, and weight machines have all been found to produce substantial increases in muscular fitness.

Similar to aerobic fitness, the ACSM has developed recommendations concerning what constitutes an appropriate resistance training protocol. An ever-increasing number of experts are recommending that older adults participate in resistance training programs for the purposes of developing musculoskeletal fitness, improving body composition, and enhancing functional capacity.

INTENSITY

The ACSM recommends that, at the minimum, an individual should perform one set of 8 to 10 exercises that train the major muscle groups. Each set should involve 8 to 12 repetitions that elicit a perceived exertion rating of 12-13* (somewhat hard). The selection of exercises should ensure that all of the major muscle groups in the body are included in the training session. Depending on an individual's personal philosophy, additional sets could be performed. Recent research conducted at the University of Florida by Pollock et al. and previous investigations at the United States Military Academy suggest that additional sets may have limited value at best.

---

* Refer to Chapter 11 for more information regarding rating of perceived exertion.

FREQUENCY

The ACSM recommends that resistance training be performed at least twice a week, with at least 48 hours of rest between workouts. Research indicates that as an individual becomes older, the need for sufficient time to recover from the resistance stress imposed upon the body increases.

DURATION

The ACSM suggests that resistance training sessions lasting longer than sixty minutes may have a detrimental effect on an individual's level of exercise adherence. Adherence to the guidelines of the ACSM would permit individuals to complete total body strength training sessions within 20-25 minutes.

Regardless of which specific protocol is adopted, several common sense guidelines pertaining to resistance training for older adults should be followed:

- Focus the major goal of the resistance training program on developing sufficient muscle fitness to enhance an individual's ability to live a physically independent lifestyle.
- Have the first several resistance training sessions be closely supervised and monitored by trained personnel who are sensitive to the special needs and capabilities of the elderly.
- Start out (the first eight weeks) with very minimal levels of resistance to allow for adaptations of the connective tissue elements.
- Teach the older participant the proper training techniques for all of the exercises to be used in the program.
- Instruct older participants to maintain their normal breathing patterns while exercising, since breath holding (i.e., performance of a Valsalva maneuver—see Appendix A) can induce excessive blood pressure elevations.
- As a training effect occurs, achieve an overload initially by increasing the number of repetitions, and then by increasing the absolute amount of resistance lifted.
- Never use a resistance that is so heavy that the exerciser cannot perform at least eight repetitions per set. Heavy resistances can be potentially dangerous and damaging to the skeletal and joint structures of an older individual.
- Stress that all exercises should be performed in a manner in which the speed is controlled. In order to prevent orthopaedic trauma to the joint structures, no ballistic (fast and jerky) movements should be allowed while exercising. Weights should be lifted and lowered in a slow, controlled manner.
- Perform the exercises in a range of motion that is within a "pain free arc" (i.e., the maximum range of motion which does not elicit pain or discomfort). As positive adaptations occur, individuals should gradually increase their exercise range of motion in order to improve their flexibility.
- Perform multi-joint exercises (as opposed to single-joint exercises) since

they tend to help individuals develop functional muscular fitness.

• Given a choice, use machines to resistance train, as opposed to free weights. The primary advantages of machines are that they tend to require less skill to use, they protect the back by stabilizing the user's body position, and they allow the user to start with lower resistances, to increase by smaller increments (this is not true for all strength training machines), and to more easily control the exercise range of motion.

• Don't overtrain. Two strength training sessions per week are the minimum number required to produce positive physiological adaptations. Depending on the circumstances, more sessions may neither be desirable nor productive.

• Never permit arthritic participants to participate in strength training exercises during active periods of pain or inflammation, since exercise could exacerbate their condition.

• Engage in a year-round resistance training program on a regular basis, since it has been shown that the cessation of resistance training can result in a rapid significant loss of strength. When returning from a lay-off, individuals should start with resistances that are equivalent to or less than 50% of the intensity at which they had been training before, and then gradually increase the resistance.

PRESCRIBING FLEXIBILITY EXERCISES

An adequate range of motion in all of the joints of the body is important to maintaining an acceptable level of musculoskeletal function. Unfortunately, efforts to identify the most effective protocol for developing flexibility (defined as the ability of the muscle, tendon, and soft tissue to yield to stretch force—a factor which, in turn, determines how much motion a skeletal joint can actually achieve) have been somewhat limited, particularly in comparison to the other basic components of physical fitness. What is almost universally accepted, but not documented, is the fact that maintaining adequate levels of flexibility will enhance an individual's functional capabilities (e.g., bending and twisting) and reduce injury potential (e.g., risk of muscle strains and low back problems)—particularly for the aged. A well-rounded program of stretching has been shown to counteract the usual decline or improve flexibility in the elderly. Not surprisingly, it is critical that a sound stretching program be included as part of each exercise session for older adults.

INTENSITY

The ACSM recommends exercises involving a slow dynamic movement, followed by a static stretch that is sustained for 10 to 30 seconds. Exercises should be prescribed for every major joint (hip, back, shoulder, knee, upper trunk, and neck regions) in the body. Three to five repetitions of each exercise should be performed. The degree of stretch achieved should not be to the point of significant pain.

FREQUENCY

The ACSM recommends that stretching exercises should be performed at least three times a week. In reality, stretching exercises should be included as an integral part of the warm-up and cool-down exercises that are performed prior to and at the conclusion of all workouts. Individuals can, however, choose to devote an entire exercise session to flexibility. This can be particularly appropriate for deconditioned older adults who are beginning an exercise program.

DURATION

The stretching phase of an individual's exercise session should involve approximately 15 to 30 minutes collectively each workout. Several common sense guidelines pertaining to stretching by older adults should be followed:

- Always precede stretching exercises with some type of warm-up activity to increase heart rate and internal body temperature. It is safer and more productive to stretch a warm muscle.
- Stretch smoothly and never bounce. When individuals bounce while stretching, they cause the muscles to tighten to protect themselves—this actually inhibits effective muscle stretching. Moreover, ballistic (i.e., bouncing) movements can cause the very sort of muscle tears that stretching is designed to prevent.
- Do not stretch a joint beyond its range of motion. Tissue has a failure point and wide variations in range of motion exist between individuals.
- Gradually ease into a stretch, and hold it only as long as it feels comfortable. If individuals stretch to the point of feeling extreme pain, they increase their likelihood of being injured.

LIVING SMART

Depending on an individual's point of reference, reflecting on the aging process may present a rather dismal picture. Certainly, many of the descriptive phrases that are often used to explain the aging process have an ominous ring to them . . . inevitable deterioration . . . negative physiological consequences . . . impaired capabilities . . . and so forth. By no means, however, is the future as bleak as it might first appear. With respect to the effects of the aging process, to a great extent, individuals can control their own destiny. Regular exercise can and does slow down many of the debilitating effects of advancing years. Irrefutable evidence exists to support the fact that mixing strict adherence to sound exercise principles with a personal commitment to common sense and patience could well serve as an appropriate recipe for improving and sustaining an independent lifestyle for the elderly. In other words, "living smart" is the fundamental priority for "living well" . . . at any age. ❏

BIBLIOGRAPHY •

1. American Dietetic Association Reports. "Nutrition, aging, and the continuum of health care." Technical support paper. *J Am Diet Assoc* 87:345-347, 1987.
2. Berger, B.G. "The role of physical activity in the life quality of older adults." *In* Spirduso, W.W., Eckert, H.M. (Eds), *The Academy Papers: Physical Activity and Aging.* Champaign, IL: Human Kinetics Publishers, 1989.
3. Bortz, W.M. "Disuse and aging." *JAMA* 248:1203-1208, 1982.
4. Bortz, W.M. "Effect of exercise on aging—effect of aging on exercise." *J Am Geriatr Soc* 28:49-51, 1980.
5. Brody, J.A., Brock, D.B., Williams, T.F. "Trends in the health of the elderly population." *Annu Rev Public Health* 8:211-234, 1987.
6. Dalsky, G.P., Stocke, K.S., Ehsani, A.A., et al. "Weight-bearing exercise training and lumbar bone mineral content in postmenopausal women." *Ann Intern Med* 108:824-828, 1988.
7. Fiatarone, M.A., Marks, E.C., Ryan, N.D., et al. "High-intensity strength training in nonagenerians: Effects on skeletal muscle." *JAMA* 263:3029-3034, 1990.
8. Fowles, D.G. *A profile of older Americans.* Program Resources Department, American Association of Retired Persons. Administration on aging, U.S. Department of Health and Human Services, 1985.
9. Frontera, W.R., Meridith, C.N., O'Reilly, K.P., et al. "Strength conditioning in older men: Skeletal muscle hypertrophy and improved function." *J Appl Physiol* 64:1038-1044, 1988.
10. Kasch, F.W., Boyer, J.L., Van Camp, S.P., Verity, L.S., Wallace, J.P. "The effect of physical activity and inactivity on aerobic power in older men (a longitudinal study)." *Phys Sportsmed* 18(4):73-83, 1990.
11. Kisner, C., Colby, L.A. *Therapeutic Exercise.* Philadelphia, PA: F. A. Davis Company, 1990.
12. Larson, E.B., Bruce, R.A. "Health benefits of exercise in an aging society." *Arch Intern Med* 147:353-356, 1987.
13. Lewis, C.B. (Ed). "Exercise and Aging." Topics in Geriatr Rehabil 1:1, 1985.
14. Morey, M.C., Cowper, P.A., Feussner, J.R., et al. "Evaluation of a supervised exercise program in a geriatric population." *J Am Geriatr Soc* 37:348-354, 1989.
15. National Center for Health Statistics. "Health, United States, 1988." DHHS Pub. No. (PHS) 89-1232. Public Health Service. Washington. U.S. Government Printing Office, March 1989.
16. Nieman, D.C. *Fitness and Sports Medicine: An Introduction.* Palo Alto, CA: Bull Publishing Company, 1990.
17. Shephard, R.J. "The scientific basis of exercise prescribing for the very old." *J Am Geriatr Soc* 38:62-70, 1990.
18. Smith, E.L., Gilligan, C. "Physical activity prescription for the older adult." *Phys Sportsmed* 11:91-101, 1983.
19. Souminen, H., Heikkinen, E., Parkitti, T. "Effect of eight weeks' physical training on muscle and connective tissue of M vastus lateralis in 69-year-old men and women." *J Gerontol* 32:33-37, 1977.
20. Spirduso, W.W., Eckhert, H. (Eds). *Physical Activity and Aging.* Champaign, IL: Human Kinetics Publishers, Inc., 1989.
21. Stanford, B.A. "Exercise and the elderly." *Exerc Sport Sci Rev* 16:341-379, 1988.
22. Work, J.A. "Strength training: A bridge to independence for the elderly." *Phys Sportsmed* 17:134-140, 1989.

CHAPTER 14

• •

ENVIRONMENTAL CONSIDERATIONS FOR EXERCISE PROGRAMS*

by

W. Larry Kenney, Ph.D.
and
Todd Crowder, Ph.D.

• • •

*U*nderstanding how your body responds and adapts to a variety of environmental conditions that can be present during exercise is critical to ensuring that you remain safe when you engage in physical activity. This chapter focuses on those specific responses and adaptations of your body to several commonly encountered environment stressors (high heat and humidity, cold, altitude, and air pollution) that affect your exercise performance capability.

HIGH HEAT AND HUMIDITY

Of the many environmental factors which can impact your opportunity to engage in safe and effective exercise, none is as potentially life—and health—threatening as heat stress. Preventing heat-related problems by properly adjusting your exercise program to account for the effects of hot ambient temperatures involves a common sense approach based on an understanding of how your body physiologically responds to heat. While few documented heat-related standards exist for recreational or clinical exercise environments, industry's experience in dealing with heat stress issues can provide important insight into such matters.

In industrial settings, heat stress has received considerable attention world-

---

* Note: Some of the material contained in this chapter is adapted from "Considerations for preventive and rehabilitative exercise programs during periods of high heat and humidity," an article which appeared in *The Exercise Standards and Malpractice Reporter* 3(1):1-7, 1989.

wide because of its potential impact on worker productivity, health, and safety. While no promulgated standard exists for heat stress evaluation and decision making, several proposed standards regarding this matter exist in the United States and across the world which provide quantitative information that can be directly applied to an exercise setting. In the U.S. alone, standards for heat stress have been proposed by the National Institute for Occupational Safety and Health (NIOSH), the American Conference of Governmental Industrial Hygienists (ACGIH), the American Industrial Hygiene Association (AIHA), and the U.S. Armed Forces. These organizations all have proposed standards aimed at preventing body temperature from rising excessively during physical exertion, mitigating the deleterious effects of dehydration, etc.. Based upon accurately assessing the environmental conditions and the intensity of physical activity, these standards can be easily adapted to an exercise setting (both indoor and outdoor). While various standards differ slightly in their approach, they typically provide two cut-off points—"action limits" above which specific actions should be taken and "ceiling limits" above which exercise should not be attempted without somehow changing the environment.

Evaluation Of The Environment

When trying to make decisions about the thermal environment, it is important that you evaluate all aspects of the environment which impact your ability to exercise safely. Not only are temperature and humidity important, but air movement and (when exercising outdoors) solar radiation also play a major role. One single temperature which takes all the effects into account is the "wet-bulb globe temperature" or "WBGT." WBGT is a single temperature index which is dependent upon air temperature, humidity, solar radiation, and wind velocity, and as a result represents a composite measure of the impact of the environment on exercising subjects.

WBGT can be measured using relatively simple low-cost instrumentation or can be calculated from data available from local weather services. Three measurements are combined into the WBGT calculation—air temperature, natural wet-bulb temperature (measured by placing a wetted wick over the thermometer bulb), and globe temperature (the temperature inside a copper globe painted flat black). Indoors, WBGT is calculated as WBGT = (0.7 x natural wet-bulb temperature) + (0.3 x globe temperature) and can be expressed as either °C or °F. Outdoor WBGT is calculated as (0.7 x natural wet-bulb) + (0.2 x globe temperature) + (0.1 x air temperature).

Basing Exercise Decisions On WBGT

It is important to remember that, even in industry, no enforced standards exist concerning heat stress. Accordingly, the recommended cut-off points presented in this section are meant to serve only as helpful guidelines in deciding such issues as "when it is too hot to exercise", "how long exercise should last under certain conditions", etc. For exercise programs and individual exercise prescription, the criteria document proposed by NIOSH [under the Occupational Safety and Health Act of 1970 (Public Law 91-596)] in 1972 and revised in 1986 can be easily adopted.

Figures 14-1 and 14-2 graphically illustrate the NIOSH's theory regarding what constitutes an appropriate approach to evaluating heat stress. Both figures define several distinct limits concerning when it is safe to exercise which are based on exercise intensity (expressed here as energy expenditure per hour) and ambient WBGT (in both °C and °F). Two sets of limits are proposed, including one set for heat-unacclimatized persons (the Recommended Alert Limit or RAL) and one for heat-acclimatized persons (the Recommended Exposure Limit or REL). Each figure also refelects a proposed "ceiling limit" (C)—a level above which probably no one should exercise unless the environment can be changed. Secondly, several action limit lines are included on each graph for intermittent exercise of varying durations.

Figure 14-1. Recommended Heat-Stress Alert Limits Heat-Unacclimatized Individuals.

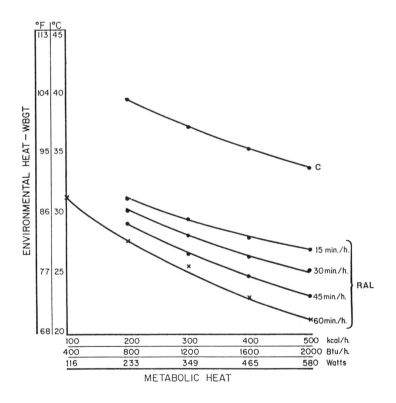

C = Ceiling Limit
RAL = Recommended Alert Limit
* For "standard individual" of 70 kg (154 lbs.) body weight and 1.8 m² (19.4 ft²) body surface.
(Based on information from DHHS NIOSH Publ. No. 86-113)

Figure 14-2. Recommended Heat-Stress Exposure Limits for Heat-Acclimatized Individuals.

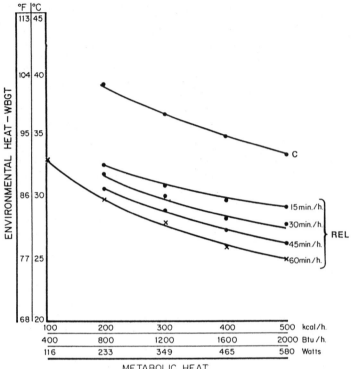

C =   Ceiling Limit
REL =   Recommended Exposure Limit
*For "standard individual" of 70 kg (154 lbs.) body weight and 1.8 m² (19.4 ft²) body surface.
(Based on information from DHHS NIOSH Publ. No. 86-113)

While it takes some practice in using such guidelines to decide when it is safe to exercise, they, in fact, provide a numerical index for making appropriate decisions about your exercise environment. Probably the most important question you may be confronted with is how to deal with an environment which is below the ceiling limit but above the RAL or REL (whichever applies). This area represents environmental conditions in which exercise can still be performed, but with an increased risk to the participant. In such cases, the following actions are recommended:

- <u>Change the environment</u>. If the exercise area cannot be cooled to an appropriate WBGT by means of fans or air conditioning, change the exercise site to one with an environment that meets the WBGT requirements;
- <u>For the session, decrease the exercise intensity</u>. Similar to cooling the environment, lowering the intensity represents another way of staying

within an acceptable temperature/intensity zone. Ways to accomplish this, while still getting a training effect, include sufficiently slowing the pace of exercise bout, adding rest cycles to a routine, etc. Perhaps the most useful technique for identifying and maintaining a safe level of exercise intensity involves the proper use of target heart rate (unchanged from cool conditions). Exercise heart rate is increased about 1 bpm for every degree Centigrade above 25 °C and 2 bpm for every mm Hg above 20 mm Hg water vapor pressure. Strict adherence to a scientifically determined target heart rate will cause an appropriate decrease in intensity.

HEAT ACCLIMATION

One of the best methods for decreasing your risk of developing a heat illness or injury is to gradually acclimate yourself to exercising in hot environments. Through this process, your heart rate and body temperature at a given exercise intensity decrease, your sweating rate increases, and your sweat becomes more dilute. It has been estimated that as much as 25% of the apparently healthy population may be heat intolerant in an unacclimated state, with that number decreasing to about 2% after thorough acclimation. The best method of acclimation is to exercise aerobically in a hot environment. The first such session may last as little as 10-15 minutes for safety reasons and gradually increase in duration to 20-60 minutes. It takes most healthy people 10-14 days to fully acclimate to hot environments, although illness and alcohol consumption have been shown to slow this process.

FLUID INTAKE

Along with heat acclimation, adequate hydration is a critical factor in preventing untoward effects of exercise when the temperature and/or humidity is high. Progressive dehydration occurs during exercise when sweating is profuse. As little as a 2% reduction in your body weight during exercise can result in impaired temperature regulation. Furthermore, a 4% decrease in body weight translates into a 6% decrease in maximal aerobic capacity and a 12% reduction in exercise time.

You should take steps to ensure that fluids are readily available so that you can drink before, during, and after exercise. All individuals should be encouraged to drink as much water as is physically comfortable 15-30 minutes prior to exercise, a cupful of water at 15 minute intervals during exercise, and more water than their sense of thirst dictates after exercise. This latter point is especially applicable if you are over the age of 60, since research has shown a decreased thirst sensitivity to body hydration status in this particular age group.

The fluid should be cold (45-55 °F) and palatable; and with a few exceptions, water is the replacement drink of choice. Little need exists to replace electrolytes lost during most exercise sessions, since these small decrements are typically replenished when the next meal is eaten. For participants on a restricted salt diet, their physician should be consulted with regard to salt balance. Unless the exercise bout lasts in excess of 90 minutes, little or no advantage can be attained by supplementing carbohydrates.

INDIVIDUALS AT RISK

The guidelines presented in this chapter are based on the assumption that the exercise participant does not have any overt disease or condition which may increase the likelihood of a heat illness or injury. Among the factors that can raise your risk of incurring heat-related problems are: hypertension (alters control of skin blood flow), diabetes (neuropathies may affect sweating and/or skin blood flow), aging (alters peripheral cardiovascular and sweating responses), various drug regimens (including diuretics, beta-blockers, alpha-agonists, and vasodilators), alcohol use (causes vasodilation and enhances dehydration), obesity, and a prior history of heat illness or difficulty acclimating to heat. It is in your best interest to be as knowledgeable as possible about the effects of each of these factors on temperature regulation (for more information refer to item 8 in the bibliography).

MANAGEMENT PLAN FOR FACILITIES

In order to be prepared to deal with real or expected periods of hot weather, personnel involved with fitness facilities should develop and implement a standardized management plan for handling stress. Among the topics which should be included in such a plan are:

1. An increase in the level of medical screening and surveillance of exercise participants.
2. An evaluation of all aspects of the facility's thermal environment, preferably using WBGT as a criterion measure.
3. An approved decision-making flowchart, concerning heat stress issues, which is based on proposed standards such as NIOSH, ACGIH, AIHA, etc., and tailored to your clientele and exercise setting.
4. A policy of strongly encouraging exercise participants to gradually acclimate to heat stress.
5. Making cold, palatable fluids readily available, and instituting a plan for increasing the fluid intake level of exercise participants before, during, and after exercise (schedule drink breaks for the entire exercise group).
6. Take steps to make exercise participants more knowledgeable about heat stress, including early signs and symptoms of heat illness (chills, light-headedness, dizziness, piloerection, nausea, etc.).
7. Emergency procedures, for handling heat illness, which have been incorporated into the overall emergency plan for the facility.

COLD

The winter months signal the advent of cold weather for most areas. Cold temperatures, however, are not an adequate reason for individuals to dramatically alter their aerobic training efforts—even if they prefer to exercise outdoors. Similar to exercising in extreme heat, you can safely exercise in the cold, provided that you adhere to a few common sense guidelines. Such guidelines are applicable to all of your alternatives for exercising aerobically outdoors in the cold, including jogging, cross-country skiing, and ice skating.

How Does the Body Respond To The Cold?

Before you identify what you personally can do to adapt to cold weather conditions, you should first consider how your body responds to the cold. Essentially, your body responds physiologically to cold weather in two primary ways: increased metabolic rate and increased tissue insulation.

Changes in metabolic rate can be elicited either voluntarily (by exercising) or involuntarily (shivering thermogenesis). Thermogenesis involves the production of heat in your body by means of shivering (and to a smaller degree, sympathetic chemical excitation). Shivering results from "cold" signals to the hypothalamus which in turn sends nonrhythmic impulses to the anterior motorneurons of the skeletal muscles throughout your body. Contrary to most individuals' perception of the process of shivering, these impulses do not cause the muscles to actually shake. Rather, they prompt the muscle spindle stretch reflex mechanism to oscillate. At a certain point, shivering begins and heat production rises. During maximal shivering, your body can increase the amount of heat it produces to as high as four to five times normal.

Before your body alters its metabolic rate, however, its initial response to the cold is to constrict blood vessels. Except for your head, this constriction occurs in the surface blood vessels in most of the peripheral areas of your body (hence the term—peripheral vasoconstriction). When blood is literally sidetracked from the surface areas of your body into the deeper blood vessels, the net effect of the process of vasoconstriction is to increase the relative insulative level of surface tissues. When blood is shunted away from a person's skin, the "insulative thickness" of the surface tissues is increased. In turn, the rate of heat loss decreases.

Exercise Responses To The Cold

Under most circumstances, cold weather should not present a significant problem for anyone who wants to exercise outdoors. Cold ambient air, for example, does not pose a particular danger to your respiratory passages. By the time that inspired air reaches the bronchi in your lungs, the air is warmed to a temperature sufficiently high to be safe. Humans can breathe air at temperatures as low as -35 °C (-31 °F) without a detrimental effect; however, in individuals who have angina, breathing cold air may interfere with their ability to recognize anginal pain. Using a scarf to cover your nose and mouth will pre-warm and pre-humidify the air.

As long as your body core temperature is kept relatively normal, and sufficient clothing is worn to keep the surface areas of your body relatively warm, your capacity to exercise will not be impaired. Your maximal ability to take in, transport, and utilize oxygen (maximal oxygen uptake) and the oxygen cost of submaximal exercise are generally unaffected by the cold. Your heart rate may be slightly lower while exercising in the cold, but this is not a universal finding. Stroke volume (the amount of blood pumped by the heart per beat) tends to be higher at low exercise intensities, but is unaffected by cold at higher workloads. Cardiac output (the amount of blood pumped by the heart on a per minute basis) is not changed.

If your core temperature and muscle temperature fall below normal, your maximal aerobic capacity and cardiovascular endurance may be reduced. A cool muscle has a decreased ability to generate force for a given cross-sectional area of muscle fibers. Therefore, in order to maintain force, more fast twitch fibers must be recruited, resulting in a greater reliance on anaerobic glycolysis and, perhaps, more lactic acid production. Thus, your ability to perform activities that require dynamic muscle strength and power may be negatively affected by cold weather.

Fortunately, the process of maintaining your body core temperature at normal levels and of insulating the exterior surface area of your body against the cold elements is not particularly difficult. As was discussed previously, under almost all conditions, your body produces sufficient heat to maintain its core temperature. Aerobic exercise makes it easier for your body to regulate its core temperature on a more voluntary basis. During exercise, more than 75% of the energy produced by your working muscles is converted to heat, which elevates core temperature. During moderate and intense exercise, sufficient heat is generated to maintain core temperature. At low intensities of exercise, however, core temperature could begin to fall after one hour of exercise in cold weather were it not for the onset of involuntary thermogenesis.

Insulating your body against the cold by wearing sufficient clothes involves common sense. Clothing traps warm air next to your skin and decreases heat loss by conduction. It is important that you wear water repellent outer clothing (to prevent soaking from rain or snow) and inner clothing which allows sweat to evaporate. Wet or damp clothing transfers heat away from your body approximately 20 times faster than dry clothing. Accordingly, the best clothing for exercising in the cold is that which protects your body from the cold, while still allowing sweat to evaporate. In recent years, significant progress has been made in the development and manufacture of cold weather exercise clothing. Clothing made of GORE-TEX™ fabric, for example, is lightweight and provides adequate protection from the environmental stressors, yet still permits water (perspiration) to evaporate.

Most experts suggest wearing several layers of clothes so that articles of clothing can be removed—a layer at a time—as you become warmer while exercising (due to increases in metabolic heat production). In general, the following guidelines are recommended with regard to clothing:

- Avoid heavy, bulky garments.
- Use up to four layers of clothing in severe weather.
- Wear an absorbent, non-irritating material for the first layer of clothing.
- Wear socks made of an absorbent, breathable material.
- Protect your hands—wear cotton or wool gloves.
- Wear a hat—large amounts of heat can be lost from an uncovered head.
- If necessary, keep your facial area warm—preferably with a wool scarf.

How Cold Is Too Cold?

Under most conditions, it will not be too cold for you to exercise outdoors provided you dress properly. In a few circumstances, however, the relative temperature will be such that exercising outdoors would be ill-advised. The most common way to express relative temperature is the wind chill index. Ambient temperature alone is not always a valid indication of "coldness." Because wind exacerbates heat loss by increasing the degree to which the warmer insulating air layer which surrounds your body is continually replaced by the cooler ambient air (collectively, it increases the convective heat loss), wind can have a substantial cooling effect on your body. For example, the combination of a -9.4 °C (15 °F) temperature with 30 MPH winds produces the equivalent temperature of -32.2 °C (26 °F). The measure used to quantify these equivalent temperatures is the wind chill index. Individuals who plan to exercise in cold weather should consult a wind chill index table (see Table 14-1) to ensure that the cooling effect of the wind—in concert with the ambient air temperature—does not place them in a potentially unsafe environment for working out. As a rule of thumb, any wind chill temperature of less than minus twenty degrees Fahrenheit should be viewed with caution and greater than minus seventy degrees Fahrenheit is potentially quite unsafe.

Table 14-1. Wind Chill Index.

Wind Speed (mph)	Thermometer reading (°F)										
	50	40	30	20	10	0	-10	-20	-30	-40	-50
	(Equivalent temperature [°F])										
5	48	37	27	16	6	-5	-15	-26	-36	-47	-57
10	40	28	16	4	-9	-24	-33	-46	-58	-70	-83
15	36	22	9	-5	-18	-32	-45	-58	-72	-85	-99
20	32	18	4	-10	-25	-39	-53	-67	-82	-96	-110
25	30	16	0	-15	-29	-44	-59	-74	-88	-104	-118
30	28	13	-2	-18	-33	-48	-63	-79	-94	-109	-125
35	27	11	-4	-20	-35	-51	-67	-82	-98	-113	-129
40*	26	10	-6	-21	-37	-53	-69	-85	-100	-115	-132

Minimal Risk	Increasing Risk	Great Risk

* Wind speeds greater than 40 MPH have little additional effect.

The key to safely exercising out-of-doors is to be prepared. Bundle up—in layers. Use common sense. Unless the wind chill index dictates otherwise, don't let the elements interfere with the benefits and joy of exercising.

ALTITUDE

The relative altitude where you exercise can also have an effect on your body. As altitude increases, barometric pressure decreases and the air becomes less dense. The percentage of oxygen in the air (20.93%) remains constant with increasing elevation, but the decrease in barometric pressure causes a reduction in the partial pressure of oxygen (pO_2). As a consequence of the reduction in pO_2, hemoglobin saturation is decreased (i.e., less oxygen is carried in the arterial blood) and the amount of oxygen available at the cellular level is diminished. This reduces maximal oxygen uptake ($\dot{V}O_2$ max), and concomitantly limits your physical working capacity (PWC). The reduction in $\dot{V}O_2$ max and PWC is directly proportional to the increase in altitude.

Changes in performance capabilities begin to manifest themselves at approximately 5,000 feet (1524 meters). For example, activities such as sprinting or long jumping tend to be enhanced at altitude—a performance improvement that likely results from the fact that your body has to overcome less resistance (since the air is less dense) while it is in flight. It appears, however, that the more aerobic an activity is, the more it will be negatively affected by altitude. As a rule, the higher the altitude, the larger the decrement in aerobic performance. Since less oxygen is present in your blood at high altitude, your heart beats more frequently to deliver a sufficient amount of oxygen to your working muscles. As a result, when you are exercising at a high altitude, you must reduce the intensity of your exercise bout in order to stay within your training heart rate range.

AIR POLLUTION

The air in most major metropolitan areas is contaminated with a variety of gases and particulates that can have a detrimental effect on exercise performance. During times of temperature inversion, or when the air becomes stagnant (i.e., air movement is low), the level of air pollutants can reach concentrations that can severely impede physical performance. The major air pollutants are carbon monoxide, ozone, and sulfur dioxide.

Carbon monoxide is an odorless gas that limits the ability of your blood to transport oxygen by binding to hemoglobin molecules (carbon monoxide has a more than 200 times greater affinity for hemoglobin than does oxygen). Exercise performance (submaximal and maximal) becomes diminished once blood concentrations of carbon monoxide reach a certain critical level (3% or greater). Ozone and sulfur dioxide both inhibit exercise performance by inducing bronchoconstriction (i.e., narrowing of the lung air passages—a process which inhibits the flow of oxygen to and from your lungs). The wheezing and coughing, characteristic of asthma, are often symptoms of overexposure to ozone and/or sulfur dioxide. Ozone has also been associated with eye irritation and nausea.

You can avoid or at least minimize the problems associated with exercising in areas of high pollution by:

- not exercising outdoors when smog alerts have been issued.
- not exercising outdoors during times when air pollutants are at their highest levels (e.g., 7-10 a.m. and 4-7 p.m.—due to heavy traffic).
- avoiding high cigarette smoking areas prior to and during exercise (carbon monoxide is a major constituent of cigarette smoke).
- not exercising outdoors when ambient temperature and humidity are high (high heat and humidity potentiate the deleterious effects of air pollution).
- reducing the amount of time spent exercising in a high pollution area (the physiological affects of air pollution are both time- and dose-dependent). ❏

BIBLIOGRAPHY •

1. Adams, W.C. "Effects of ozone exposure at ambient air pollution episode levels on exercise performance." *Sports Med* 4:395-424, 1987.
2. American Conference of Governmental Industrial Hygienists. "Threshold limit values for chemical substances and physical agents in the workroom environment with intended changes." ACGIH, Cincinnati, 1979.
3. American Industrial Hygiene Association. "Heating and cooling for man in industry," 2nd Ed. AIHA, Akron, 1975.
4. Balke, B. "Variations in altitude and its effects on exercise performance." *In* Falls, H. (Ed), *Exercise Physiology*. New York, NY: Academic Press, pp. 240-265, 1968.
5. Brooks, G.A., Fahey, T.D. *Exercise Physiology: Human Bioenergetics and Its Applications.* New York, NY: John Wiley & Sons, 1984.
6. Hage, P. "Air pollution: adverse effects on athletic performance." *Phys Sportsmed* 10:126-132, 1982.
7. Horvath, S.M. "Exercise in a cold environment." *Exerc Sport Sci Rev* 9:221-263, 1981.
8. Kenney, W.L. "Physiological correlates of heat intolerance." *Sports Med* 2:279-286, 1985.
9. National Institute for Occupational Safety and Health. "Criteria for a recommended standard...occupational exposure to hot environments." (DHHS NIOSH Publ. No. 86-113), U.S. Department of Health and Human Services, Washington D.C., 1986.
10. Pierson, W.E., Covert, D.S., Koenig, J.Q., et al. "Implications of air pollution effects on athletic performance." *Med Sci Sports Exerc* 18:322-327, 1986.
11. Powers, S.K., Howley, E.T. *Exercise Physiology: Theory and Application to Fitness and Performance.* Dubuque, IA: Wm. C. Brown Publishers, 1990.
12. Sawka, M.N. et al. "Hydration and vascular fluid shifts during exercise in the heat." *J Appl Physiol* 56:91-96, 1984.
13. Sutton, J.R., Jones, N.L. "Exercise at altitude." *Ann Rev Physiol* 45:427-437, 1983.
14. Triservices Document. "Prevention, treatment, and control of heat injury." *US Army TB Med* 507, 1980.

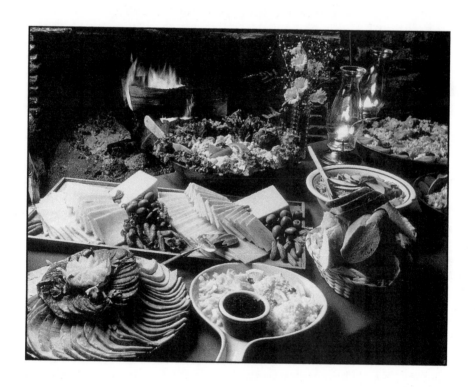

CHAPTER 15

· ·

NUTRITIONAL CONSIDERATIONS FOR EXERCISE

by

Karol J. Fink, B.S.
and
Bonnie Worthington-Roberts, Ph.D.

• • •

Nutrition can play a substantial role in almost every aspect of your life. Since inadequate nutrition can have a negative affect on your ability to engage in most of the tasks attendant to daily living, good nutrition is absolutely essential. Good nutrition involves providing your body with the required nutrients in appropriate amounts. Each distinct nutrient performs special functions that other nutrients cannot. Synergistically, the nutrients depend upon each other to provide the energy your body needs. Accordingly, obtaining all of the essential nutrients from food each day is especially important for you to be able to participate in physical activity programs.

The essential nutrients are grouped into two main categories—each with three separate entities. The nutrients without calories are water, vitamins and minerals; while the caloric nutrients are carbohydrates, protein and fat. The nutrients with calories supply the energy you require to perform your daily living activities. As such, they are particularly important during exercise. Although, the non-caloric nutrients do not directly provide energy, they have an essential role because they participate in energy-producing reactions. Without their presence, your body could not produce energy.

HOW TO OBTAIN ADEQUATE AMOUNTS OF EACH NUTRIENT

Proper nutrition is an extremely important component of a sound training regime. When mapping out a workout schedule for the week, nutrition should be included. While sound nutritional practices will not convert a mediocre athlete into an Olympian, they will provide the requisite nutritional ingredients for enabling individuals to enhance their capability to perform at their (genetically determined) best.

News articles, friends, restaurants, physicians, dietitians, coaches, and trainers often refer to the terms "proper," "good," and "balanced" nutrition. Despite such a focus on nutrition, understanding what the words "proper," "good," or "balanced" nutrition really mean and how to attain proper nutrition is a frequently confusing undertaking.

A simple way to ensure that your body's nutrient needs are being met is to understand and adhere to the Four Food Group model, which was developed to aid the American public in attaining proper nutrition. Most American elementary schools use the Four Food Group model for educating students about nutrition. As a result, it is quite likely that most athletes and exercisers have had some exposure to the concept. The major benefit of the Four Food Group model is that it can be easily understood and integrated into the daily dietary habits of most people.

The four groups in this model are the:

• meat and high protein group
• milk and dairy product group
• cereals and grain group
• fruit and vegetable group

Foods are classified into a particular group because of their vitamin and mineral content, as well as their carbohydrate, protein, and fat content. The Federal Government has established recommendations concerning how many servings from each group you should eat on a daily basis (refer to Table 15-1). Meeting these recommendations will adequately supply all of the essential vitamins and minerals required for an individual leading an active lifestyle (with the possible exception of the minerals iron and calcium). Although eating the recommended servings of the four food groups will ensure that all the essential vitamins and minerals an individual needs are supplied in adequate quantities, satisfying the recommendations will not necessarily ensure that every individual will be provided with an adequate level of caloric intake.

Your caloric requirements depend upon specific individual characteristics (e.g., age, gender, height, and weight), as well as specific program variables (e.g., the type, frequency, intensity, and duration of the regimen in which you participate). Most exercisers will require more calories than the minimum recommended number of servings will provide. A healthy way exercisers can obtain the extra calories they need is to increase the serving sizes of foods from both the cereal and grain group and the fruit and vegetable group, and the amount of non-animal high protein foods they eat.

Table 15-1. Recommended minimum number of servings from the Basic Four Food Groups with serving sizes.

Food Group	Recommended minimum number of servings			
	Teenagers	Adults	Pregnant women	Lactating women
Meat	2	2	3	2
Milk	4	2	4	4
Fruit-vegetable	4	4	4	4
Bread-cereal	4	4	4	4

Serving sizes

Meat: one serving is
2 ounces cooked, lean, boneless meat, fish, poultry or protein equivalent
2 eggs
2 slices (2 oz) cheddar cheese *
1/2 cup cottage cheese *
1 cup cooked dry beans, peas, lentils or soybeans
1 cup nuts
4 tablespoons peanut butter

Milk: one serving is
1 cup milk, yogurt, or calcium equivalent
1 slice (1-1/2 oz) cheddar cheese *
2 ounces processed cheese food *

Fruit-vegetable: one serving is
1/2 cup cooked or juice
1 small salad
1 orange
1/2 cantaloupe
1 medium potato

Bread-cereal: one serving is
1 slice bread
1 cup (1oz) ready-to-eat cereal
1/2 cup cooked cereal or pasta

* A serving of cheese can be used or either milk or meat group, but not both

Modified from Williams, M.H. (1988).

WHAT DOES EACH FOOD GROUP HAVE TO OFFER?

The cereal and grain group is an excellent source of carbohydrates, both complex and simple. It is also a good source of protein, vitamins, and minerals—particularly thiamin (B_1), iron (due to fortification), and niacin. Among the foods which are included in this group are breads, breakfast cereals, pastas, rice, tortillas, and taco shells. Foods that are made from oats, flour, or corn meal, such as pancakes or corn bread, are also included in the grain and cereal group.

The fruit and vegetable group provides many important vitamins and minerals. The composition of nutrients in different fruits and vegetables is extremely varied. For this reason it is important to select different fruits and vegetables throughout the week. In general, the fruit and vegetable group is an excellent source of the key vitamins A and C and also provides a good general supply of most other vitamins and minerals. Some fruits and vegetables that are particularly healthy choices are broccoli, spinach, carrots, bananas, and oranges.

Cheese, yogurt, cottage cheese, ice cream, and milk are all included in the milk and dairy product group. These foods not only are an excellent source of protein, but they also provide several important vitamins and minerals. Calcium is the most common mineral associated with this group, because milk and dairy products are the greatest contributor of calcium in the typical American diet. Calcium plays a vital role in the growth and maintenance of bones and teeth. It is important that you consume the recommended minimum amount of milk and dairy product servings each day, because your reliance upon calcium for the maintenance of healthy bones and teeth continues throughout your life.

The meat and high protein group supplies protein, niacin, iron, zinc, and thiamin. These nutrients are important for the maintenance of muscles, bones, red blood cells (the oxygen carrying component of blood), and healthy skin. Foods which are classified in this group include eggs, beef, pork, chicken, fish, luncheon meats, tuna, and hot dogs. Examples of high protein non-animal foods include legumes (beans), nuts, and peanut butter. These foods are included in the meat and high protein group because of their high protein and key nutrient content. Limiting your consumption of animal products to a moderate level—one to two servings a day—is recommended because such foodstuffs are commonly high in saturated fat and cholesterol. Choosing high protein, non-animal foods more often than animal products is recommended because such foods provide a greater variety of nutrients (including carbohydrates and fiber) and contain no cholesterol.

A fifth group, the "others" category, is often mentioned during discussion of the Four Food Group model. This group encompasses foods lacking in nutrients, such as alcohol, fats and oils, sweets, chips, crackers, soft drinks and condiments. Foods in the "others" category typically are high in calories, high in fat, high in sodium (salt), and low in beneficial nutrients. Foods from the "others" category should only be eaten after ensuring that the minimum number of recommended servings of each food group has been met in your diet. The "other" foods should only be eaten in moderation, as an adjunct to an already healthy balanced diet.

How To Evaluate A Day's Meals Using The Four Food Groups

The Four Food Group classification provides a straightforward and simple way to evaluate food intake and determine if your nutrient needs are being met. Evaluating the food intake of an individual based on the Four Food Groups involves keeping a record of the amount of all food and beverage consumed throughout the day. This record is then compared to what is recommended (refer to Table 15-2). If the recommended number of servings from a certain group is not ingested, the individual may not be acquiring an adequate amount of nutrients. Knowing the actual serving size will enable you to be better able to determine if your nutritional needs are being met. For example, one cup of milk constitutes a full serving of the milk and dairy product group, while two cups of cottage cheese is considered a serving.

A thorough evaluation of the sample one-day diet record illustrated in Table 15-2 indicates that this person did not consume enough calcium or riboflavin (the individual only had one dairy product serving) and had not ingested a substantial amount of vitamins and minerals. This particular shortcoming, for example, could have been supplied by two more servings of fruits and vegetables. To avoid intake deficiencies in the future, this individual could make dietary changes that might include choosing milk instead of a cola at lunch, eating a piece of fruit for a midday snack and eating a vegetable serving with dinner. Changes such as these are relatively small yet helpful ways which the individual can undertake to ensure that adequate amounts of all nutrients are ingested.

Table 15-2. Evaluation of a one-day diet record based on the Four Food Groups.

Food	Amount	Grain & Cereal	Fruit & Vegetable	Milk & Dairy	Meat & Protein	"Others" Group
Bran Flakes	1.5 cups	2				
Banana	1 medium		1			
Milk, 1%	1 cup			1		
Whole Wheat bread	2 slices	2				
Luncheon Meat	2 slices				1 (animal)	
Mayonnaise	1 tbsp.					1
Cola	1 can					1
Spaghetti	1 cup	2				
Tomato & Meat Sauce	1/2 cup 2 ounces		1		1 (non-animal)	
French Bread	1 slice	1				
Beer	1 can					1
TOTAL		7	2	1	2	3
Recommended amount		4	4	2	2	0
Serving difference		+3	-2	-1	0	+3

REDEFINING THE BASIC FOUR FOOD GROUPS

A new concept, the "Food Pyramid," has recently been developed and endorsed by the United States Department of Agriculture (1992) to replace the basic four food groups. Although this graphically illustrated pyramid has not been fully adopted or developed, its use is expected to begin in the near future—replacing the Four food group model. The message of the food pyramid is not much different than that of the four food group model. Both recommend approximately the same number of servings. The fundamental difference between the two models is distinguished by the emphasis of bread, cereals, rice, pasta, vegetables and fruits and the de-emphasis of animal and dairy products.

Since a pyramid cannot exist without a foundation, the bottom layer is built with breads, cereal, rice, and pasta to depict the relative importance of these foods. The pyramid recommends a varied combination (9-11 servings) for these foods each day. For its building materials, the second layer of the Pyramid relies upon vegetables (3-5 servings each day) and fruits (2-4 servings each day). The construction materials for the third layer are contained in two equal compartments. One of meat, poultry, fish, beans, eggs, and nuts (2-3 servings), and the other of milk, yogurt and cheese (2-3 servings). Although this layer is smaller and attempts to de-emphasize the use of animal products, the number of servings recommended is equal to or greater than that of the four food group model. The very small apex of the pyramid contains fats, sweets, alcohol, and oil—foods that you should consume in extremely limited amounts.

The food pyramid is based on a recommendation that you consume a minimum daily number of servings from each of the six food categories every day. It also is predicated on the suggestion that you focus more on building a strong, balanced foundation by emphasizing breads, cereals, rice, pasta, vegetables, and fruit as the major portion of your diet. As you continue to build your personal pyramid, you should eat a variety of foods that result in a strong, balanced, healthy diet.

Figure 15-1. The Food Guide Pyramid.

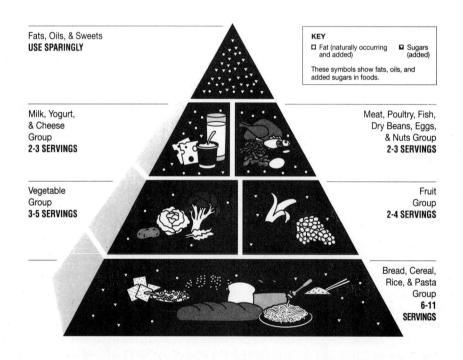

CARBOHYDRATE

Most physically active individuals realize they should eat a diet rich in carbohydrates. Although they may know this, they often do not realize why this is important, or even of what a diet rich in carbohydrates would consist. Carbohydrates are an important means of replenishing your glycogen stores. Glycogen is your muscles' preferred source of fuel during aerobic exercise, because it is efficiently converted to energy. The availability of glycogen has been shown to influence the amount of exercise you can accomplish before fatigue occurs. This section of the chapter presents an explanation of the relationship between carbohydrate and glycogen, describes the importance of glycogen during exercise, and offers suggestions for increasing your dietary intake of carbohydrates.

GLYCOGEN AND CARBOHYDRATES AS FUEL

Carbohydrates are composed of complex and/or simple sugars that are readily converted into glucose once they are absorbed into the blood. The amount of glucose in the blood is strictly regulated to ensure that tissues dependent on blood glucose energy (e.g., the brain, heart and kidneys) have a constant supply of fuel. If your blood glucose concentration rises (as it does after eating carbohydrates), the excess glucose is stored as glycogen in your liver and muscles. Once your glycogen storage capacity has been met, the excess glucose is converted and stored as fat.

Blood glucose and liver glycogen are easily interconverted in your body because glycogen is made from linking glucose molecules together. If your blood glucose concentration decreases, glucose molecules are broken off from liver glycogen and reenter the blood stream. This control mechanism prevents large fluctuations in blood glucose levels from occurring and ensures that your dependent tissues are constantly supplied with energy.

Similar to liver glycogen, muscle glycogen is constantly utilized over the course of a day. Whereas liver glycogen supplies energy to organs and tissues, muscle glycogen provides energy exclusively to your working muscles. Muscle glycogen provides the best source of fuel during aerobic exercise because it is simply and readily converted to energy. Fat and protein are able to provide energy during exercise, but the process of their conversion to energy is much more complex than that of glycogen. The easy conversion of glycogen to energy helps optimize performance by decreasing the amount of work your body must do to produce energy.

The supply of muscle glycogen during vigorous exercise can last from 60 to 90 minutes depending on how much of this energy source was stored in your muscles prior to the onset of exercise. The amount of glycogen you store depends upon your level of daily carbohydrate and calorie replenishment and your level of fitness. As a general rule, the better trained an individual is, the more glycogen an individual can store. A non-exercising individual, who eats a proper diet and participates in normal daily activities, will not experience a depletion of muscle glycogen during a typical day even though muscle glycogen is constantly being used. Engaging in normal daily activities, as well as prolonged or intense exercise, however, will result in the greater utilization of glycogen for fuel, thereby depleting your glycogen stores. Exercisers have termed this depletion "hitting the wall" or "bonking" because it correlates with fatigue and exhaustion.

Low or depleted muscle glycogen stores at the onset of aerobic exercise, or glycogen stores that become low or depleted during exercise, can cut your workout short due to premature fatigue and exhaustion caused by a lack of sufficient fuel. Low or depleted muscle glycogen stores can limit the intensity at which you can exercise, or result in a tired and listless feeling the remainder of the day, or until your muscle glycogen stores are replenished. No exerciser wants to experience the symptoms of low or depleted muscle glycogen stores that can result in a compromised workout, or influence the outcome of a competition. Consequently, ensuring a sufficient intake of dietary carbohydrates should be a paramount concern of the physically active individual.

DIETARY CARBOHYDRATES

Your body must convert dietary carbohydrates into glycogen, because dietary glycogen does not exist. Since a single workout lowers your muscle glycogen stores, a daily intake of a sufficient amount of calories and carbohydrates is essential for the replenishment of muscle glycogen stores. Carbohydrates are found in a wide variety of foods in the form of starches and simple sugars. Starches are complex carbohydrates which exist in many foods. The grain and cereal food group, which includes foods such as bread, pasta, rice, cereals, and grains, is a good source of complex carbohydrates. Beans, peas, and certain vegetables (e.g., potatoes and corn) are also good sources of complex carbohydrates. Simple sugars are found in a variety of foods. In most instances, they provide the "sweet" flavor found in foods. Examples of nutritious foods containing simple sugars include fruit, fruit juices, and milk. In contrast, several foodstuffs from the "others" food group, such as sodas, sweet baked products, ice cream, chocolate, candies, and foods prepared with refined white sugar or honey, represent non-nutritious simple sugars..

Even though such products are high in simple sugars (which are carbohydrates), they are not the most appropriate choice for glycogen replacement. Consuming foods rich in simple sugars prior to working out can disturb your body's strict balance of blood glucose. Simple sugars are absorbed quickly into the bloodstream, causing a rapid increase in blood glucose. This increase, in turn, activates your body's mechanisms for regulating blood glucose levels so quickly that your blood glucose levels may actually swing too low. Interfering with this complex regulatory system may result in your having an inadequate level of fuel during exercise. For this reason, it is usually suggested that simple sugars should not be eaten for several hours prior to exercise. Complex carbohydrates, on the other hand, do not have the same impact on blood glucose as simple sugars. Complex carbohydrates are absorbed more slowly into your blood, thereby minimizing the risk of undesirable fluctuations in blood glucose levels. They also supply several important nutrients which are usually lacking in foods containing simple sugars.

INCREASING DIETARY CARBOHYDRATE

Each time you exercise, you are utilizing and relying upon stored muscle glycogen for fuel. This process results in lowered muscle glycogen storage at the end of a workout. Consuming a carbohydrate-rich diet will replenish your glycogen supplies to ensure adequate and/or optimal glycogen storage. Adopting a daily meal pattern rich in complex carbohydrates is the best way to replenish and maintain your glycogen stores. To increase the amount of complex carbohydrates in your diet, you should eat more servings from the cereal and grain food group, in addition to eating more beans and vegetables. These complex carbohydrate-rich foods efficiently replenish your glycogen stores and provide you with several other important nutrients.

Nutritious foods which are high in simple sugars, such as fruit, fruit juices and milk, are a much better choice than most "other" simple sugar rich foods. These foods not only provide nutrients, but their carbohydrate makeup is less likely to result in undesirable fluctuations in your blood glucose levels. For example, the simple sugars contained in milk and fruit are absorbed and converted to blood glucose quicker than complex carbohydrates. Foods high in simple sugars, however, are absorbed and converted to blood glucose more slowly than are the aforementioned examples of the sugar-laden "other" foods. Therefore, fruit, fruit juices, and milk provide a good source of carbohydrate to replenish your glycogen supplies. Animal foods from the meat and high protein food group contain little or no carbohydrates. As a result, it is very difficult to replenish your glycogen stores by eating steak, poultry, or fish. Several examples of carbohydrate-rich food choices are presented in Table 15-3.

Table 15-3. Carbohydrate-Rich Food Choices.

Complex	Not-So Nutritious Simple Carbohydrates
Bread, rolls, bagels, and English muffins (especially whole grain)	Products made with refined white sugar or honey
Whole grain breakfast cereals, pancakes, and corn bread	Sweet baked products, cookies, and cakes
Rice, brown, white, long or short grained	Sweetened fruit juices
Vegetables (especially potatoes and corn)	Ice cream and frozen yogurt
Cooked beans and peas	Chocolate and candy bars
Pasta and noodles	Carbonated beverages
Nutritious Simple Carbohydrates	
Fruits and non-sweetened fruit juices	
Dried fruits	
Milk	

By more frequently choosing complex carbohydrate and nutritious simple carbohydrate foods, or by substituting these choices for foods in the "others" category, you can easily increase the amount of daily dietary carbohydrates that you consume. You can increase the likelihood that you will have a diet which is high in complex carbohydrates by undertaking certain steps, including:

- Consuming a varied diet containing the recommended amount of servings from each food group.
- Consuming several additional servings from the cereal and grain group.
- Consuming extra fruits and vegetables in order to ensure that you ingest a sufficient level of calories.

PROTEIN

In recent years, many athletes have begun to better understand the fact that the role of dietary carbohydrate is more important as an energy source than dietary protein. This realization is not based on the assumption that protein is unimportant, but rather that as a fuel source during exercise, protein appears to have a very limited role.

Dietary protein is essential for many functions within your body. For example, it is a major component of muscle. It also serves as a structural basis for all of the enzymes and hormones which control the basic physiological functions in your body. It helps maintain the proper hydration level in your body. Finally, when needed, protein can act as a source of energy. Considering the important role protein plays in human functioning, consuming an adequate level of dietary protein is essential for all individuals—including athletes. The question arises, however, concerning whether an athlete or a physically active individual needs to consume more protein-rich foods than a sedentary person.

UNDERSTANDING PROTEIN RECOMMENDATIONS

The Recommended Daily Allowance (RDA) for protein provides a standard designed to ensure good nutrition for a healthy American adult and is based on the minimum daily amount of protein required for proper maintenance of body tissue. Since variability exists between individuals, the RDA recommendation includes a "safety factor" to ensure that almost all healthy people will be covered by this umbrella recommendation. The RDA for protein is 0.8 grams per kilogram (2.2 pounds) of body weight. This recommendation is basically useless for anyone besides an exercise scientist, physician, or registered dietitian. It is, however, what most researchers base their studies and conclusions on for determining if athletes require more protein. Most studies in this area have attempted to answer the question: "Do athletes require more protein than the RDA of 0.8 grams per kilogram body weight?" This is not a "user friendly" question for the general population. Even though the RDA for protein exists, individuals are unaware of the recommendation and would typically not know how to incorporate it into their lives, even if they were exposed to the RDA guideline for protein.

An analysis of the existing literature on the protein requirements of physically active individuals suggests that it would be more appropriate for such research to focus instead on the questions: "How much protein do athletes eat now?" and "Are they meeting their current needs for protein?" It appears that the data obtained by answering these two questions would be more applicable to the athletic population than the conclusions current research provides. National food consumption studies indicate that most Americans consume 1.5 to 2 times the RDA for protein. Specific studies calculating the actual dietary protein intakes of athletes have found intakes greater than 1.5 to 2 times the RDA. Comparison of what would be thought to be two extremes, football players and female ballet dancers, reveals similar results. The football players were shown to consume well over 2 times the RDA for protein, while the ballet dancers ingested greater than 1.5 times the RDA for protein.

Thus, even if the recommendation for the athlete may be greater, the average individual and the athlete are already consuming enough protein to ensure proper levels of consumption. One reason most exercisers are exceeding the RDA recommendation is because they have high caloric intakes. When more calories are consumed from a varied diet, increases in all nutrients occur—including protein. So even if active individuals require more protein, they are most likely already meeting the needs of their bodies.

PROTEIN FOODS

Foods in each of the four food groups provide protein (refer to Table 15-4). Obviously, the meat and high protein food group tends to provide the largest amounts of protein. Foods from the milk and dairy product group and cereal and grain group also supply an ample amount of protein. Fruits provide a relatively insignificant amount of protein to the diet. On the other hand, vegetables are a relatively good source of protein. According to the RDA, a 130-pound (59 kilogram) woman should consume 47 grams of protein daily, while a 154-pound (70 kilograms) man should consume 56 grams. This amount of protein (and more) can easily be provided by a varied, well-balanced diet, consisting of foods from each food group.

HOW MUCH PROTEIN DO ATHLETES REALLY REQUIRE?

Two issues should be addressed when discussing the protein needs of an athlete: protein as a source of fuel, and protein for building muscle mass. Research conducted in the early 1800s surmised that since muscles include considerable protein, then protein must be the preferred fuel for muscles and that increases in muscle mass must come from extra dietary protein. It is now known that carbohydrate, in the form of muscle glycogen, contributes the primary fuel for muscle. It is also known that training is what builds and strengthens muscles, not simply extra dietary protein.

Even though scientists agree that protein is not the primary fuel or cause of increased muscle mass, they believe that protein plays an important secondary role during exercise that may increase an athlete's need for protein above the RDA. The American Dietetics Association's (ADA) most recent report on sports and nutrition recommended increased protein requirements only for individuals involved in intense aerobic training (greater than 70% VO_2 max). Even though ADA made the recommendation, it recognizes that the average American, including an athlete, consumes protein above this recommendation. The ADA does not support the notion that the protein needs of a competitive weight lifter are greater—all of the dietary protein a weight lifter may need is provided from a well-balanced diet. An individual who would like to add muscle bulk should focus on combining a sound resistance training program with a well-balanced diet.

Most scientists and dietitians agree that exercise does not increase the body's need for protein significantly. A few, however, believe that physically active

Table 15-4. Protein Content of Selected Foods.

FOOD	PROTEIN (grams)
Meat & High Protein Group	
Tuna, canned, drained 4 oz.	31.0
Chicken, 1/4 Ib. cooked	31.0
Hamburger, 1/4 Ib. cooked	31.0
Sirloin steak, 1/4 Ib. cooked	27.0
Egg, 1 medium	6.0
Soybeans, 1/2 cup cooked	12.0
Peanut butter, 1 tbsp.	7.0
Most beans, 1 cup cooked	15.0
Milk & Dairy Product Group	
Milk, 1 cup	9.0
Cottage Cheese, 1/2 cup	14.0
Cheese, 1 slice	7.0
Ice cream, 1/2 cup	3.0
Yogurt, plain 1 cup	11.0
Cereal & Grain Group	
Spaghetti, 1 cup cooked	6.0
Rice, brown, 1 cup cooked	5.0
Rice, white, 1 cup cooked	4.0
Bread, 1 slice	3.0
Bagel, 1 whole	6.0
Fruit & Vegetable Group	
Broccoli, 1/2 cup cooked	2.0
Carrots, 1 large	1.0
Corn, 1 ear	4.0
Green peas, 1/2 cup cooked	4.0
Apple, 1 medium	0.3
Banana, 1 medium	1.0
Grapes, 1 cup	0.5

individuals have an increased need for protein. Peter Lemon, Ph.D., professor of applied physiology laboratory at Kent State University, is one the most renowned advocates of the theory of an increased protein need for athletes. He recommends that athletes should consume between 1 to 1.5 times more protein than the established RDA. Since the average American, including an athlete, already consumes 1.5 to 2 times the RDA, it would appear as though athletes need not to increase their protein intake.

ARE THERE ANY RISKS ASSOCIATED WITH EXCESS PROTEIN CONSUMPTION?

Your body is unable to store extra protein. Protein consumed in excess of your body's needs is not used to build muscle but used for nonprotein bodily functions. If you consume protein in excess of your caloric and protein needs, the extra protein will not be stored as protein but converted to and stored as fat. As a result, if you consume large amounts of extra protein in addition to your regular diet, any weight gain would very likely be in the form of fat.

Potential for harm exists if protein is consumed in excess. The results are most likely to occur in the individual who consumes protein or amino acid supplements. Excess protein may lead to dehydration, because protein metabolism requires extra water for utilization and excretion (i.e., elimination) of its by-products. Since exercising individuals are already at an increased risk for dehydration (refer to the fluid balance section of this chapter), the additional strain of protein waste excretion may further encourage dehydration. Excess protein has also been shown to lead to an increase in the loss of urinary calcium. A chronic calcium loss, due to excess protein intake, is of particular concern because it increases the risk of osteoporosis, especially in women.

Young man's death raises question of safety

A healthy, athletic 23-year old male university student died of anaphylactic schock allegedly due to the body building amino acid supplement he ingested. Anaphylactic shock, caused by a severe allergic reaction to an allergen, is rare, but other mild allergic reactions to body building amino acid supplements may be common. One manufacturer of amino acid supplements previously claimed that their supplement "won't trigger common food allergies." The amino acid supplement this young man took did not trigger a common allergy, it triggered one that may have ended his life. It is advisable to avoid such protein and amino acid supplementation since the benefits of supplementation are yet undetermined, in addition to the fact that single amino acid supplements have not been thoroughly tested in human subjects, and, therefore, no margin of safety is available.

DIETARY FAT AND CHOLESTEROL

Research indicates that a diet high in fat and cholesterol can increase your risk for atherosclerosis (narrowing of the arteries), heart disease, and certain types of cancer. Atherosclerosis results when excess fat and cholesterol are deposited within your arteries, narrowing the passage for blood to flow through. If the passage becomes too narrow and blood flow is reduced significantly, anginal chest pain or a heart attack can occur. Decreasing the amount of dietary fat and cholesterol reduces your risk of coronary heart disease, aids in losing weight and increases the carbohydrate percentage in your diet.

BLOOD CHOLESTEROL

Two concepts should be understood when discussing cholesterol: blood cholesterol and dietary cholesterol. Blood cholesterol, measured by a clinician and expressed in milligrams per deciliter (mg/dl), is a factor which helps identify an individual's risk for heart disease. Dietary cholesterol is found only in foods of animal origin. As a preventive measure against the development of a high level of blood cholesterol, your dietary intake of cholesterol should be limited to less than 300 milligrams per day.

Although high blood cholesterol has harmful effects, cholesterol plays a vital and necessary role in proper human functioning. Cholesterol is involved in hormone production, cell wall structure development, and digestion. The amount of cholesterol in your blood is influenced by proper liver function, dietary cholesterol intake, exercise, body weight, and other yet to be identified influences. Problems arise when the concentration of cholesterol in your blood reaches unhealthy levels (refer to Table 15-5). When your blood cholesterol level reaches a certain point, the risk of harmful cholesterol and fat deposits forming in your arteries rises, increasing your chances of developing cardiovascular disease.

Table 15-5. Risk Classification Based on Total Cholesterol.

TOTAL CHOLESTEROL READING	CLASSIFICATION
<200 mg/dl	Desirable Blood Cholesterol
200-239 mg/dl	Borderline-High Blood Cholesterol
> or = 240 mg/dl	High Blood Cholesterol

Persons over the age of 20 should have their blood cholesterol levels checked at least once every five years. An annual recheck of blood cholesterol levels above 200 mg/dl is recommended. For individuals with cholesterol levels greater than 200 mg/dl, it is recommended that dietary changes, exercise, and lifestyle changes be the first measures adopted to help lower cholesterol levels. It is important that at-risk individuals consult with the proper health professionals before initiating any lifestyle or dietary changes for blood cholesterol reduction.

INFLUENCING BLOOD CHOLESTEROL WITH DIET AND EXERCISE

To avoid high blood cholesterol and its complications, adopting dietary preventive measures and exercising are top priorities. Adopting a low-fat diet with its prudent limitation of how much eggs, beef, pork, and other animal products you eat has been shown to be the best way for individuals to decrease the cholesterol content of their diets. One serving of an animal product per day from the meat and high protein food group, plus the avoidance of high fat processed foods and the consumption of nonfat or low-fat milk and dairy products, will help ensure that your dietary cholesterol intake is appropriately low. Engaging in an exercise program on a regular basis which adheres to the accepted exercise guidelines (refer to chapter 11) also has been found to produce desired changes in blood cholesterol profiles.

LIMITING DIETARY FAT

The American Heart Association recommends limiting your intake of dietary fat to less than 30% of your total calories. Most average Americans consume greater than 35% of their total calories from fat. One half of this dietary fat comes from animal products such as red meat (beef, pork, lamb, veal), poultry, fish and shellfish, separated animal fats (products fried in tallow or lard), dairy products (milk and cheese), and eggs. Some other contributors of fat in the diet include salad dressings and oils, most convenience foods, sweet baked products, and confections. Much of the fat and cholesterol we obtain is hidden in the foods we eat. Identifying foods high in fat and cholesterol is the key way to learn how to avoid them. Cholesterol is only found in animal foods and products. If an animal product is high in fat, it is usually high in cholesterol. As a general rule, meats and meat products and most processed and prepared foods—potato chips, crackers, frozen meals, cakes, and cookies—are high in fat. Tables 15-6 and 15-7 provide the calorie, cholesterol and percent fat of some common foods and note healthy low fat and low cholesterol alternatives (marked by *) to these choices.

Prepared foods, even though they are not animal products, can contain cholesterol depending on the type of fat or ingredient used. For example, potato chips fried in lard will contain cholesterol, while chips fried in vegetable shortening will not. It is important to note, however, that both these foods would be high fat, since they were fried. Baked goods made with eggs (cakes and cookies) contain cholesterol from the egg yolk and are generally high fat due to the butter, margarine, or oil included in the recipe. Whole milk and dairy products can also be high in fat and cholesterol. Alternative low-fat and nonfat products containing less fat and cholesterol, however, are available. Fresh and frozen fruits and vegetables (exceptions include avocados, coconuts, and olives) contain only small amounts of fat and should not be limited in an effort to reduce dietary fat intake.

The typical active American adult should limit the amount of dietary fat consumed both as a preventive health measure and a possible performance enhancer. A decrease in your consumption of fat will usually result in a healthy low-fat diet. A low-fat diet (less than 30% of calories coming from fat) is typically

Table 15-6. Calorie, Cholesterol, and Fat Content of Selected Foods.

Food	Amount	Calories	Cholesterol (mg)	% Fat
Fried Chicken	breast	260	95	75
Big Mac	1	570	85	55
Fried Fish	3 oz.	194	69	51
Steak	3 oz.	250	83	54
Baked Chicken*	breast	220	84	45
Baked Chicken w/out skin*	breast	175	85	20
Broiled Fish*	3 oz.	90	47	<1
Egg, whole	1 large	80	272	68
Egg, yolk only	1 large	63	272	80
Egg, white only*	1 large	16	0	0
Egg, substitute*	1/4 cup	96	1	66
Doughnut	1	105	0	34
Bran Muffin (small)*	1	100	0	27
Toast (dry)*	1 slice	80	0	7
Bagel (not egg)*	1	160	0	1
Granola	1/4 cup	125	0	29
Oatmeal*	3/4 cup	105	0	17
Bran Flakes*	3/4 cup	95	0	<1
Guacamole	1/4 cup	100	0	95
Salsa*	1/4 cup	10	0	0
Potato Chips	1 oz.	150	0	60
Peanuts	1 oz.	165	0	76
French Fries	1 pkg.	160	0	51
Chocolate Bar	1 bar	250	6	50
Tortilla Chips*	1 oz.	150	0	48
Popcorn (unbuttered)*	1 cup	25	0	<1
Apple (small)*	1 piece	60	0	0
Banana*	1 piece	90	0	0
Cream	1 tbsp.	37	13	97
Nonfat Evaporated Milk*	1 tbsp.	13	<1	<1
2% Milk	1 cup	125	18	36
Nonfat Milk*	1 cup	90	5	<1
Potato with Sour Cream	1 medium	270	10	17
Plain Potato*	1 medium	100	0	0
Butter	1 tbsp.	100	33	100
Margarine*	1 tbsp.	100	0	100
Clam Chowder	1 cup	165	22	38
Chicken Soup*	1 cup	75	3	60
Beer	12 oz.	145	0	0
Wine	3.5 oz.	72	0	0
Soda	12 oz.	150	0	0
Diet Soda	12 oz.	1	0	0

* These are wiser choices of foods that the preceding one(s).

Table 15-7. Percent Fat Found in Common Foods.

	Fruits & Vegetables	Cereal & Grain	Milk & Dairy	Meat and High Protein Group			Combination & "Others" Foods
				Legumes & Nuts	Poultry & Fish	Red Meat	
Low in fat <15% of calories coming from fat	Fruits: fresh frozen, canned, dried Plain vegetables (no added fat) Pure fruit juices	Grains & flours: barley, rice, corn, wheat, most breads & breakfast cereals bagels, pita bread, corn tortillas, noodles & pasta	Nonfat (skim): milk, yogurt, cottage cheese	Dried beans & peas: garbanzo, lima, pinto, black, kidney, split peas, lentils, black-eyed	Egg whites, cod, flounder, perch, haddock, perch, tuna (in water), shrimp, scallops	Completely trimmed: beef (round, tips, flank), pork, luncheon meats 0-2 grams fat/oz. (turkey 97% fat free, ham 94% fat free)	Spaghetti with tomato sauce, mustard, soy sauce, catsup, sherbert, juice bars, soft drinks
Medium in fat 15-30% of calories from fat		Corn bread, flour tortillas, soft rolls & buns, wheat germ, soda crackers	Low fat: yogurt, cottage cheese		Light meat of chicken and turkey (without skin), turkey breast, bass, catfish, crab, clams, fresh tuna, lobster	Completely trimmed: beef (round, tips, flank), pork, luncheon meats 0-2 grams fat/oz. (turkey 97% fat free, ham 94% fat free)	Frozen "diet" meals, beans in tomato sauce, animal cookies, ginger snaps, graham crackers, ice milk, frozen low fat yogurt
High in fat 30-50% of calories coming from fat		Biscuits & muffins, granola cereals, pancakes & waffles, snack crackers	Low fat milk (2%), most reduced calorie cheese, ice milk	Soybeans, tofu	Light meat of chicken & turkey (with skin), dark (without skin), turkey luncheon meats, salmon, tuna drained of oil, albacore	Completely trimmed: beef, veal, lamb, ham, Canadian bacon	Fish sticks, burritos, most frozen meals, hamburgers, pizza, spaghetti with meat, macaroni & cheese, french fries, cakes, candy bars, cookies, granola bars, doughnuts, ice cream
Very high in fat >50% of calories coming from fat	Avocado, olives, coconut	Snack chips, croissants, pastries	Whole milk, most cheeses, nondairy creamers, half & half, cream, ice cream	Most nuts & seeds, peanuts and peanut butter	Dark meat of chicken and turkey (with skin), whole eggs, ground turkey, anchovies, trout, tuna in oil	Partially trimmed meats: Beef, veal, lamb, pork, spareribs, ground beef, bacon, sausages, most luncheon meats, hot dogs	Fried chicken, hot dogs, onion rings, potato chips, snack chips, nachos, cream soups, mayonnaise, salad dressing, chocolate, "gourmet" ice creams, butter, margarine.

Adapted from "Eating for a Healthy Heart," American Heart Association, Alameda County Chapter.

high in carbohydrates, fruits and vegetables, fiber, vitamins and minerals—all of which benefit an individual who exercises (since it helps maintain adequate levels of glycogen). A list of suggestions regarding how you can lower the amount of dietary fat you consume is discussed in Table 15-8.

LABEL READING FOR FAT AND CHOLESTEROL

Label reading to determine the fat content of food can be quite a tricky process. Labels can read 97% Fat Free, low fat, reduced fat, less fat, lean, lite, light, etc., and still be laden with fat. The wide array of label terminology confuses the consumer who often purchases products based on the label's claim regardless if it is truly lower in fat or not. An easy way to determine if a product is high in fat is to read the ingredients listed on the label. If a fat, oil, shortening, or meat is listed near the beginning or if several different fats are listed, then the product is generally high in fat.

The American Heart Association's recommendation that less than 30% of your calories should come from fat is far different from what labels frequently claim in their advertising text. To more accurately determine the amount of fat in a product, referring to the nutritional information on the label panel is most beneficial. Hopefully, this panel lists the number of calories and grams of fat per serving. By using these two numbers, the percent of fat contained in that food can be calculated. For example, a 2-ounce slice of luncheon meat which is labeled "80% Fat Free" derives more than half of its calories from fat:

Example of Label	
"80% Fat Free Luncheon Meat"	
Serving size	2 oz.
Calories	145
Fat (g)	10
Carbohydrate (g)	0
Protein (g)	14

The number of fat grams should be multiplied by nine (because fat supplies nine calories per gram) to convert the fat grams to calories. The resultant number is then divided by the total number of calories to calculate the percent of calories from fat:

$$\frac{\text{Fat (g) x 9 calories per gram of fat}}{\text{Number of calories}} = \text{the percent of calories derived from fat}$$

For the aforementioned example of "80% Fat Free Luncheon Meat"

$$\frac{\text{10 g of fat x 9 calories per gram of fat}}{\text{145 calories}} = \text{62 percent calories from fat}$$

This "80% Fat Free" product derives 62% of its calories from fat. The average consumer would expect the product to contain 20% fat because of the "80% Fat Free" claim (80% + 20% = 100%). However, "80% Fat Free" represents the percent fat free per unit weight which is different from the percent of calories. The American Heart Association's recommendation of less than 30% dietary fat is based on calories, not weight. Thus, this "80% Fat Free" product is far greater than the 30% or less recommendation and would be considered high in fat. Label reading is essential to avoid the confusion caused by the deceptive claims of food manufacturers.

Definitions for the claims manufacturers make are not consistent from product to product because two different federal agencies regulate the terminology. The United States Department of Agriculture (USDA) supervises labels on meat products, most poultry products and eggs, while the Food and Drug Administration (FDA) supervises most other foods. Some overlap of which agency is responsible occurs. In addition, some foods are regulated by the state in which they are sold. With different agencies regulating different products, it seems impossible to know what the claim on the label really means. Among the definitions of some common food label terms and the respective agency responsible for regulating the use of a specific term are the following:

• *Leaner/Lower Fat/Less Fat (USDA)*
  May be used if there is at least a 25 percent reduction in fat content as compared to the original product.

• *Lite/Light/Lightly (FDA & USDA)*
  USDA policy indicates these terms may be used if there is a 25 percent reduction in fat as compared to the original meat or poultry product. These words are commonly used to refer to calories and sodium, and the same 25% reduction guidelines can be applied. FDA policy, which regulates the use of these terms, is somewhat meaningless, because few standards exist. These policies are deceiving to the consumer, especially with a product such as "extra light" olive oil. This claim refers to the color and extraction method used; it has nothing to do with a reduction in calories or fat.

• *Low Calorie (FDA & USDA)*
  Products containing no more than 40 calories per serving; be sure to determine if the serving size is reasonable.

• *Low Fat (FDA)*
  Refers to most milk and dairy products. The product must have a fat content by weight of less than 2% (for low fat milk, this is still 35% of its calories from fat).

• *Low Fat/Lean/Extra Lean (USDA)*
  These terms can be used on meat and poultry products (except ground beef and hamburger) that are not more than 10% fat by weight. The term "extra lean" may be used when a product is no more than 5% fat by weight (except

ground beef and hamburger). For ground beef and hamburger, the terms "lean" and "extra lean" require the product to be less than 22.5% fat by weight, compared to regular ground beef at 30% fat by weight.

• *No Cholesterol or Cholesterol Free (FDA)*
Food contains less than two milligrams cholesterol and no more than 5 grams total fat per serving.

• *Low Cholesterol (FDA)*
Food contains fewer than 20 milligrams of cholesterol per serving and no more than 5 grams total fat per serving.

• *Reduced Cholesterol (FDA)*
Foods must have at least a 75% reduction in cholesterol from the original product. The amount of cholesterol in the original and improved product must be listed.

Table 15-8. How to Make a "Fat" Difference in Your Diet.

---

1. **Read the labels.** Check the serving size on the nutritional label, and then identify the number of grams of fat per serving. Compare brands, and select the product with the least amount of fat.

2. **Limit your intake of added fats.** Butter, Margarine, salad dressings, and cooking oils have about 10 grams of fat per tablespoon. Use a low-fat or a non-fat substitute instead. Many reduced-fat commercial products are currently on the market.

3. **Eat lean meats.** Substitute lower-fat cuts of meat for those high in fats. Ask your butcher for advice if needed.

4. **Eat poultry instead of read meat.** Chicken and turkey usually have less fat than beef or pork. Poultry-based luncheon meats and ground meat are also lower in fat than their beef and pork counterparts.

5. **Trim and skin your meat.** Remove all visible fat from meat and poultry prior to cooking. Also, remove the skin from poultry.

6. **Limit your portions of meat.** Limit your intake of meat and poultry to less than three ounces per serving—six ounces per day.

7. **Eat more fish.** Most fish are lower in fat, especially saturated fat, than are red meats and poultry.

8. **Eat water-packed tuna.** Tuna packed in water has substantially less fat and calories than oil-packed.

9. **Eat low-fat frozen dinners.** If you eat frozen dinners, buy frozen dinners that have a maximum of 10 grams of fat per serving; some frozen dinners have as few as six to seven grams of fat.

10. **Eat low-fat dairy products.** Be heart-healthy selective when eating all dairy products. For example, use non-fat (skim) milk or 1% milk instead of whole or 2%. Use non-fat or low-fat yogurt instead of whole-milk yogurt or sour cream. Eat non-fat frozen desserts instead of ice cream. If you eat cheese, eat cheese that has less than five grams of fat per ounce.

11. **Eat vegetable protein foods.** Dry beans and peas are low in fat and high in both protein and soluble fiber (which reduces your blood cholesterol level).

12. **Limit your intake of nuts and seeds.** Although nuts and seeds have protein and fiber, both are high in fat.

13. **Eat complex carbohydrates.** Replace foods high in fat with non- or low-fat starchy foods such as pastas, whole-grain breads, rice, vegetables, and cereals.

14. **Eat fruits and vegetables.** Eat at least five to six servings a day of fruit and vegetables—both are high in essential vitamins, minerals, and fiber.

15. **Eat low-fat breads and cereals.** Some breads (e.g., croissants) and cereals (e.g., granola) are high in fat (often saturated fat). Read the label and select low-fat alternatives (e.g., bagels) accordingly.

16. **Limit your intake of fried foods.** Eat foods that have been baked, broiled, grilled, poached, steamed, microwaved, or roasted instead of fried. Battered and breaded foods that have been deep-fried are very high in fat.

17. **Use vegetable coating sprays.** Coat your non-stick skillet with a vegetable spray instead of oil, butter, or margarine.

18. **Use unsaturated fats for cooking.** Unsaturated fats (monounsaturated and polyunsaturated) are found primarily in vegetable oils (such as peanut, olive, canola, sunflower, and corn). Replacing unsaturated fats for saturated fats has been found to reduce cholesterol levels in some individuals.

19. **Limit your intake of sauces and gravies.** Most sauces and gravies should be avoided because they are made with fat. Instead, eat natural juices, fat-skimmed broth, and vegetable salsas.

20. **Limit your intake of chocolate.** Substitute cocoa, which has less fat, for chocolate.

Unfortunately, the existing terminology for labeling is not particularly helpful when trying to select foods which are low in fat and cholesterol. Reading the list of ingredients is the first step to determining if a product is low in fat. The next step is to calculate the actual percentage of fat using the equation which was discussed earlier in this section. In general, if less than 30% of a food's calories are from fat, it is considered to be a good choice. This does not mean a food with greater than 30% of its calories coming from fat should never be eaten. Rather this food should be eaten in moderation or with a low-fat food to balance out the total fat percentage of your diet.

WEIGHT MANAGEMENT

Approximately 25% of the adult American population is considered to be obese. Yet, more than 50% of American adults feel they have a weight problem. Billions are spent annually on diet books, diet pills, diet drinks, etc. We live in a weight-conscious society that has produced people who are willing to try almost anything to lose weight. Unfortunately, the commonly employed methods of weight loss tend not to be either physiologically sound or safe.

Weight loss occurs when an individual is in a negative caloric balance. A negative caloric balance can be achieved by either reducing calorie intake through dietary measures or increasing caloric expenditure through physical activity. Weight loss that occurs only by severe calorie restriction can result in the break-down of muscle tissue for energy and limited amounts of fat loss. The less muscle tissue you have, the lower your metabolic rate will be. Thus, the more weight individuals lose through dieting alone, the more their metabolic rates will decline and the greater their tendency to regain the weight they have lost.

Weight charts are commonly used to provide individuals with an idea of what an appropriate weight might be for them. Yet body composition, as measured by percent fat, is a much better indicator of whether you need to lose weight. As a result, a weight chart should only be used as a guide to what you should weigh—not as an absolute ideal. For example, a six-foot male weight lifter who has only 8% body fat, yet weighs 230 pounds due to his large amount of muscle mass, would be considered to be (at a minimum) 40 pounds overweight according to standard height-weight charts. In fact, however, the man would, in all likelihood, be extremely fit and should not consider losing weight to merely fall within a reference weight range.

It is important to keep in mind that weight gain does not occur in a day or a week. Accordingly, it is not realistic to expect weight loss to occur that quickly. The combination diet-exercise approach to weight reduction tends to produce a rate of weight loss of about one to two pounds per week (the rate of weight loss recommended by most experts), meaning it will take you longer to reach your desired goal. Statistics indicate, however, that weight which is lost in this manner is much less likely to be regained.

DIETARY CHANGES FOR WEIGHT MANAGEMENT

Extremely restricted diets, whether they involve dietary regimens that strictly control caloric intake, liquid diets or diets in which the consumption of only a few types of food is allowed, should be avoided due to the potentially harmful effects they can have on your body. The fundamental basis for a sound diet should begin with meeting the minimum number of servings recommended by the Four Food Group model. This guideline ensures that you will consume a minimum level of calories and nutrients each day. Once the base dietary pattern following the Four Food Groups has been established, individuals with higher caloric needs can add additional servings and still lose weight. High calorie foods do not have to be eliminated from your diet completely. Eating smaller portion sizes or consuming high calorie food less often will make any dietary modifications easier to incorporate into your lifestyle. Reducing the total amount of fat in your diet is another worthwhile dietary strategy for weight reduction.

Dietary fat intake is of primary concern for anyone desiring to lose weight since fat contains nine calories per gram, while carbohydrates and proteins only contain four calories per gram. For example, switching from 2% milk to nonfat milk results in a calorie savings of 35 calories per cup due to the elimination of fat. It becomes quite clear that reducing dietary fat will have a significant effect upon your ability to reduce the total number of calories that you consume.

WHY IS EXERCISE IMPORTANT?

Exercise is the only reasonably safe and effective method for increasing caloric expenditure. An individual can expect to burn 200-300 calories during a 30-minute bout of moderately intense aerobic exercise (refer to chapter 11 for more detailed exercise prescription information). In addition, exercise has been shown to help individuals maintain their amounts of lean tissue and possibly their resting metabolic rates. A recent survey published in the American Journal of Clinical Nutrition revealed that 90% of maintainers (individuals who lose weight and keep it off) exercise on a regular basis, while only approximately one-third of relapsers (individuals who lose weight only to regain it) were physically active. Rather than simply promoting immediate weight loss, exercise helps to ensure that weight loss is permanent. Finally, it is important to remember that exercise can greatly improve your health regardless of its effect on body composition. ❏

BIBLIOGRAPHY •

1. Berning, J.R., Steen, S.N. (Eds). Sports Nutrition *for the 90s: The health professional's handbook.* Gaithersburg, MD: Aspen Publishers, Inc., 1991.
2. Clark, N. "Fueling up with carbs: How much is enough?" *Phys Sportsmed* 19(8):68-69, 1991.
3. Franklin, B.A., Rubenfire, M. "Losing weight through exercise." *JAMA* 4:244, 1980.
4. Lemon, P.W.R. "Protein and exercise: Update 1987." *Med Sci Sports Exerc* 19(5):S179-S190, 1987.
5. Marcus, J. *Sports Nutrition, Sports and Cardiovascular Nutritionists.* Chicago, IL: The American Dietetics Association, 1986.
6. McCathy, P. "How much protein do athletes really need?" *Phys Sportsmed* 17(5):170-175, 1989.
7. Pennington, J.A.T. *Food values of portions commonly used.* New York, NY: Harper & Row, 1989.

8. Slavin, J.L., Lanners, G., Engstrom, M.A. "Amino acid supplements: Beneficial or risky?" *Phys Sportsmed* 16(3):221-224, 1988.
9. Smith, N.J., Worthington-Roberts, B. *Food for sport*. Palo Alto, CA: Bull Publishing Company, 1989.
10. Whitney, E.N., Hamilton, E.M.N. *Understanding Nutrition*, 4th Ed. New York, NY: West Publishing Company, 1987.
11. Williams, M.H. *Nutrition for fitness and sport*, 2nd Ed. Dubuque, IA: Wm. C. Brown Publishers, 1988.

EPILOGUE

· ·

TEN GUIDELINES FOR SENSIBLE EXERCISE

1. *Define your exercise goals.* Identify what you expect to accomplish from your exercise program (e.g., improve aerobic fitness, lose weight, improve upper body muscular fitness, etc).

2. *Engage in a sound exercise regimen.* Base your exercise prescription on scientifically-based information, for example, on the guidelines developed by the American College of Sports Medicine.

3. *Focus on safety at all times.* Be sensitive to the need for safety. For example, you should obtain appropriate clearance before initiating an exercise program; adhere to established exercise guidelines; err on the side of conservatism whenever in doubt—particularly when beginning your program; and properly use all exercise equipment (refer to Appendices C and D).

4. *Assess your overall fitness level.* Evaluate how fit you are before starting your exercise program and at periodic intervals (e.g., approximately every six months) thereafter.

5. *Strive for total fitness.* Include activities for all the components of health-related fitness—cardiorespiratory fitness, muscular fitness, body composition, and flexibility—in your exercise program.

6. *Eat sensibly.* Keep in mind that a sound nutrition program goes hand-in-hand with a sound exercise regimen.

7. *Do not overtrain.* Avoid doing too much, too hard, too soon (refer to Appendix E for a listing of the common signs or symptoms of overtraining)—keep in mind that exercise is not a contest; the primary goal of your exercise program should be to enable you to achieve the objectives which are important to you.

8. *Record your training progress.* Keep a detailed record of your exercise efforts. Such a record can serve several purposes, including allowing you to accurately evaluate the effectiveness of your exercise program on an on-going basis (refer to Appendix F for sample exercise recording forms); helping to motivate you; providing you with a "status" report; etc.

9. *Make exercise a habit.* Establish a pattern of exercising on a regular basis—you'll receive the greatest benefits in your health and fitness level when you make exercise an integral part of your lifestyle.

10. *Make your exercise program enjoyable.* Select activities that you enjoy—if you like what you're doing, you will substantially increase the likelihood that you will adhere to the program.

APPENDIX A

· ·

GLOSSARY OF SELECTED
FITNESS TERMS

· ·

A GLOSSARY OF
SELECTED FITNESS TERMS*

(Note: This glossary includes an overview of words pertaining to exercise, health, medicine, nutrition, physiology, etc.)

Acclimation
A program undertaken to induce acclimatization to new environmental conditions such as changes in temperature or altitude.

Acclimatization
The body's gradual adaptation to a changed environment, such as higher temperatures or lower pressures (from high altitude).

Acute
Sudden, short-term, sharp or severe. Cf. chronic

Adaptation
The adjustment of the body (or mind) to achieve a greater degree of fitness to its environment. Adaptations are more persistent than an immediate response to the new stimuli of the environment. Cf. response.

Adherence
Sticking to something. Used to describe a person's continuation in an exercise program. Cf. compliance.

Adipose tissue
Fat tissue.

Aerobic
Using oxygen.

Aerobic activities
Activities using large muscle groups at moderate intensities that permit the body to use oxygen to supply energy and to maintain a steady state for more than a few minutes. Cf. steady state.

Aerobic endurance
The ability to continue aerobic activity over a period of time.

Aerobic power
See maximal oxygen uptake.

Agonist
A muscle which directly engages in an action around a joint which has another muscle that can provide an opposing action (antagonist).

Amino acids
The building blocks of protein. Twenty different amino acids are required by the body. Cf. essential amino acids.

Anabolic
Pertaining to the putting together of complex substances from simpler ones, especially to the building of body proteins from amino acids.

Anabolic steroids
A group of synthetic, testosterone-like hormones that promote anabolism, including muscle hypertrophy. Medical uses include promotion of tissue repair in severely debilitated patients, but their use in athletics is considered unethical and carries numerous serious health risks.

---

* Adapted from Fitness Management Products & Services Source Guide. 8(3): 195-206, 1992.

Anabolism

The process of combining simple substances to build living matter by the cells. For example, combining amino acids into proteins to build muscle cells. Cf. catabolism, metabolism.

Anaerobic

Not using oxygen.

Anaerobic activities

Activities using muscle groups at high intensities that exceed the body's capacity to use oxygen to supply energy and which create an oxygen debt by using energy produced without oxygen. Cf. oxygen.

Anaerobic endurance

The ability to continue activity over a period of time (much shorter time than with aerobic activity).

Anaerobic threshold

The point where increasing energy demands of exercise cannot be met by the use of oxygen, and an oxygen debt begins to be incurred.

Anatomy

The science of the structure of the human body.

Anemia

A subnormal number or hemoglobin content of red blood cells caused when blood loss exceeds blood production. Symptoms may include fatigue, pale complexion, light headedness, palpitations, and loss of appetite.

Angina

A gripping, choking, or suffocating pain in the chest (angina pectoris), caused most often by insufficient flow of oxygen to the heart muscle during exercise or excitement. Exercise should stop, and medical attention should be obtained.

Anorexia

Lack of appetite. Anorexia nervosa is a psychological and physiological condition characterized by inability or refusal to eat, leading to severe weight loss, malnutrition, hormone imbalances, and other potentially life-threatening biological changes.

Antagonist

A muscle that can provide an opposing action to the action of another muscle (the agonist) around a joint.

Anthropometry

The science dealing with the measurement (size, weight, proportions) of the human body.

Aquatics

Exercise or sports activities in or on the water.

Arrhythmia

Any abnormal rhythm of the heart beat. Since some causes of arrythmia may have serious health consequences, exercisers experiencing irregular heart beats should be referred for medical evaluation.

Arteriosclerosis

Thickening and hardening of the artery walls by one of several diseases. Cf. atherosclerosis.

Artery

Vessel which carries blood away from the heart to the tissues of the body.

Arthritis

Inflammation of the joints which causes pain, stiffness and limitation of motion. May be symptomatic of a systemic disease, such as rheumatoid arthritis, which can affect all age groups. Cf. osteoarthritis.

Atherosclerosis

A very common form of arteriosclerosis, in which the arteries are narrowed by deposits of cholesterol and other material in the inner walls of the artery. Cf. arteriosclerosis.

Atrophy

Reduction in size, or wasting away, of a body part, organ, tissue or cell. Cf. hypertrophy.

Ballistic movement

An exercise movement in which part of the body is "thrown" against the resistance of antagonist muscles or against the limits of a joint. The latter, especially, is considered dangerous to the integrity of ligaments and tendons.

Basal metabolic rate

The minimum energy required to maintain the body's life function at rest. Usually expressed in calories per hour per square meter of body surface. Cf. met.

Biofeedback

A process which permits a person to see or hear indicators of physiological variables, such as blood pressure, skin temperature, or heart rate, which may allow the person to exert some control over those variables. Often used to teach relaxation techniques.

Blood pressure

The pressure exerted by the blood on the wall of the arteries. Maximum and minimum measures are used: The systolic pressure reaches a maximum just before the end of the pumping phase of the heart; the diastolic pressure (minimum) occurs late in the refilling phase of the heart. Measures are in the millimeters of mercury (as 120/80). Cf. hypertension.

Body composition

The proportions of fat, muscle, and bone making up the body. Usually expressed as percent of body fat and percent of lean body mass.

Body density

The specific gravity of the body, which can be tested by underwater weighing. Compares the weight of the body to the weight of the same volume of water. Result can be used to estimate the percentage of body fat.

Bradycardia

Slow heart beat. A well-conditioned heart will often deliver a pulse rate of less than 60 beats per minute at rest, which would be considered bradycrotic by standard definitions. Cf. tachycardia.

Bursa

A cushioning sac filled with a lubricating fluid that alleviates friction where there is movement between muscles, between tendon and bone, or between bone and skin.

Bursitis

The inflammation of a bursa, sometimes with calcification in underlying tendon.

Calisthenics

A system of exercise movements, without equipment, for the building of the strength, flexibility and physical grace. The Greeks formed the word from "kalos" (beautiful) and "sthenos" (strength).

Calorie cost

The number of Calories burned to produce the energy for a task. Usually measured in Calories (kcal) per minute.

Calorie

The Calorie used as a unit of metabolism (as in diet and energy expenditure) equals 1,000 small calories, and is often spelled with a capital C to make that distinction. It is the energy required to raise the temperature of one kilogram of water one degree Celsius. Also called a kilocalorie (kcal).

Capillary

The tiny blood vessels that receive blood flow from the arteries, interchange substances between the blood and the tissues, and return the blood to the veins.

Carbohydrate

Chemical compound of carbon, oxygen and hydrogen, usually with the hydrogen and oxygen in the right proportions to form water. Common forms are starches, sugars, cellulose, and gums. Carbohydrates are more readily used for energy production than are fats and proteins.

Carbon dioxide

A colorless, odorless gas that is formed in the tissues by the oxidation of carbon, and is eliminated by the lungs. Its presence in the lungs stimulates breathing.

Cardiac

Pertaining to the heart.

Cardiac output

The volume of blood pumped out by the heart in a given unit of time. It equals the stroke volume times the heart rate.

Cardiac rehabilitation

A program to prepare cardiac patients to return to productive lives with a reduced risk of recurring health problems.

Cardiopulmonary resuscitation (CPR)

A first-aid method to restore breathing and heart action through mouth-to-mouth breathing and rhythmic chest compressions. CPR instruction is offered by local Heart Association and Red Cross units, and is a minimum requirement for most fitness-instruction certifications.

Cardiorespiratory endurance

See aerobic endurance.

Cardiovascular

Pertaining to the heart and blood vessels.

Carotid Artery

The principal artery in both sides of the neck. A convenient place to detect a pulse.

Catabolism

The process of breaking down complex substances into simpler parts by the cells. For example, breaking down carbohydrates or fats for use in energy expenditure. Cf. anabolism, metabolism.

Cellulite

A commercially created name for lumpy fat deposits. Actually this fat behaves no differently from other fat; it is just straining against irregular bands of connective tissue.

Cholesterol

A steroid alcohol found in animal fats. This pearly, fatlike substance is implicated in the narrowing of the arteries in atherosclerosis. Plasma levels of cholesterol are considered normal between 180 and 230 milligrams per 100 milliliters. Higher levels are thought to pose risks to the arteries.

Chronic

Continuing over time.

Circuit training

A series of exercises, performed one after the other, with little rest between. Resistance training in this manner increases strength while making some contribution to cardiovascular endurance as well. (It remains controversial as to whether a significant cardiovascular benefit will be achieved in the absence of very consistent motivation or close supervision of the sessions).

Collateral circulation

Blood circulation through small side branches that can supplement (or substitute for) the main vessel's delivery of blood to certain tissues.

Compliance

Staying with a prescribed exercise program. (Often used in a medical setting.) Cf. adherence.

Concentric action

Muscle action in which the muscle is shortening under its own power. This action is commonly called "positive" work, or, redundantly, "concentric contraction." Cf. eccentric action, isometric action.

Concussion

An injury from a severe blow or jar. A brain concussion may result in temporary loss of consciousness and memory loss, if mild. Severe concussion causes prolonged loss of consciousness and may impair breathing, dilate the pupils and disrupt other regulatory functions of the brain.

Conditioning

Long-term physical training.

Connective tissue

A fibrous tissue that binds together and supports the structures of the body. Cf. fascia, joint capsules, ligament, tendon.

Contraindication

Any condition which indicates that a particular course of action (or exercise) would be inadvisable.

Cool down

A gradual reduction of the intensity of exercise to allow physiological processes to return to normal. Helps avoid blood pooling in the legs and may reduce muscular soreness.

Coronary arteries

The arteries, circling the heart like a crown, that supply blood to the heart muscle.

Coronary heart disease (CHD)

Atherosclerosis of the coronary arteries.

Cross-sectional study

A study made at one point in time. Cf. longitudinal study.

Defribrillator

A device used to stop weak, uncoordinated beating (fibrillation) of the heart and allow restoration of a normal heart beat. Part of the "crash cart" at cardiac rehabilitation program sites.

Dehydration

The condition resulting from the excessive loss of body water.

Detraining

The process of losing the benefits of training by returning to a sedentary life.

Diastole

Relaxation phase of the heart. Cf. systole.

Diastolic blood pressure

The minimum blood pressure that occurs during the refilling of the heart. Cf. blood pressure.

Diet

The food one eats. May or may not be a selection of foods to accomplish a particular health or fitness objective.

Diuretic

Any agent which increases the flow of urine. Used inadvisedly for quick weight loss, diuretics can cause dehydration.

Dry-bulb thermometer

An ordinary instrument for indicating temperature. Does not take into account humidity and other factors that combine to determine the heat stress experienced by the body. Cf. wet-bulb thermometer, wet-globe temperature.

Duration

The time spent in a single exercise session. Duration, along with frequency and intensity, are factors affecting the effectiveness of exercise.

Dyspnea
Difficult or labored breathing.

Eccentric action
Muscle action in which the muscle resists while it is forced to lengthen. This action is commonly called "negative" work, or "eccentric contraction," but, since the muscle is lengthening the word "contraction" is misapplied. Cf. concentric action, isometric action.

Efficiency
The ratio of energy consumed to the work accomplished. Exercisers utilizing the same amounts of oxygen may differ in their speed or amount of weight moved in a given time because of differing efficiencies.

Electrocardiogram (EKG, ECG)
A graph of the electrical activity caused by the stimulation of the heart muscle. The millivolts of electricity are detected by electrodes on the body surface and are recorded by an electrocardiograph.

Electrolyte
A substance which, in solution, is capable of conducting electricity. Certain electrolytes are essential to the electrochemical functioning of the body.

Endurance
The capacity to continue a physical performance over a period of time. Cf. aerobic endurance, anaerobic endurance.

Energy
The capacity to produce work.

Epidemiological studies
Statistical study of the relationships between various factors that determine the frequency and distribution of disease. For example, such studies have linked exercise to reduced mortality.

Epiphyseal plates
The sites of new bone growth, separated from the main bone by cartilage during the growth period. This is a potential injury site to be avoided in prescribing exercise to prepubescent individuals.

Epiphyses
The ends of long bones, usually wider than the shaft of the bone.

Ergometer
A device that can measure work consistently and reliably. Stationary exercise cycles were the first widely available devices equipped with ergometers, but a wide variety of endurance-training machines now have ergometric capacity.

Essential amino acids
Those amino acids that the body cannot make for itself. They are: isoleucine, leucine, lysine, methionine, phenylalanine, tryptophan, and valine.

Essential hypertension
Hypertension without a discoverable cause. Also called primary hypertension. Cf. hypertension.

Estrogen
The sex hormone that predominates in the female, but also has functions in the male. It is responsible for the development of female secondary sex characteristics, which have an effect on female responses to exercise. Cf. testosterone.

Exercise
Physical exertion of sufficient intensity, duration, and frequency to achieve or maintain fitness, or other health or athletic objectives.

Exercise prescription
A recommendation for a course of exercise to meet desirable individual objectives for fitness. Includes activity types, duration, intensity, and frequency of exercise.

Exercise program director

Certification as exercise program director by the American College of Sports Medicine indicates the competency to design, implement, and administer preventive and rehabilitative exercise programs, to educate staff in conducting tests and leading physical activity, and to educate the community about such programs. Must have all the competencies of the certified fitness instructor, exercise test technologist, and exercise specialist.

Exercise specialist

A person certified by the American College of Sports Medicine as having the competency and skill to supervise preventive and rehabilitative exercise programs and prescribe activities for patients. Must also pass the ACSM standards for exercise test technologist.

Exercise technologist

A person certified by the American College of Sports Medicine as competent to administer graded exercise tests, calculate the data, and implement any needed emergency procedures. Must have current CPR certification.

Expiration

Breathing air out of the lungs. Cf. inspiration, respiration.

Extension

A movement which moves the two ends of a jointed body part away from each other, as in straightening the arm. Cf. flexion.

Extensor

A muscle that extends a jointed body part.

Faint

See syncope.

Fascia

Connective tissue which surrounds muscles and various organs of the body.

Fast-twitch fibers

Muscle fiber type that contracts quickly and is used most in intensive, short-duration exercises, such as weightlifting or sprints. Cf. slow-twitch fibres.

Fat

1. A white or yellowish tissue which stores reserve energy, provides padding for organs, and smooths body contours. 2. A compound of glycerol and various fatty acids. Dietary fat is not as readily converted to energy as are carbohydrates.

Fat-free weight

Lean body mass.

Fatigue

A loss of power to continue a given level of physical performance.

Fitness

The state of well-being consisting of optimum levels of strength, flexibility, weight control, cardiovascular capacity and positive physical and mental health behaviors, that prepare a person to participate fully in life, to be free from controllable health-risk factors and to achieve physical objectives consistent with his/her potential. Cf. wellness.

Fitness center

A place furnished with space and equipment, where leadership and supervision are offered to further the fitness objectives of participants.

Fitness Instructor

A person who directs classes or individuals in the performance of exercise. Certification by the American College of Sports Medicine indicates the competency to identify risk factors, conduct submaximal exercise tests, recommend exercise programs, lead classes, and counsel with exercisers. Works with persons without known disease. CPR certification is required.

Fitness testing

Measuring the indicators of the various aspects of fitness. Cf. graded exercise test, physical work capacity.

Flexibility

The range of motion around a joint.

Flexion

A movement which moves the two ends of a jointed body part closer to each other, as in bending the arm. Cf. extension.

Foot-pound

The amount of work required to lift one pound one foot.

Frequency

How often a person repeats a complete exercise session (e.g. 3 times per week). Frequency, along with duration and intensity, affect the effectiveness of exercise.

Functional capacity

See maximal oxygen uptake.

Glucose

Blood sugar. The transportable form of carbohydrate, which reaches the cells.

Glycogen

The storage form of carbohydrate. Glycogen is used in the muscles for the production of energy.

Golgi tendon organ

Organs at the junction of muscle and tendon that send inhibitory impulses to the muscle when the muscle's contraction reaches certain levels. The purpose may be to protect against separating the tendon from bone when a contraction is too great. Cf. muscle spindle, proprioceptor.

Graded exercise test (GXT)

A treadmill, or cycle-ergometer, test that delivers heart rate, ECG, and other data. Workload is gradually increased until an increase in workload is not followed by an increase in oxygen consumption; this identifies the individual's maximal oxygen uptake. Allows the prescribing of exercise to the individual's actual, rather than estimated, heart rate or aerobic capacity. Requires medical supervision. Cf. physical work capacity.

Growth hormone

Human growth hormone (HGH), somatotrophin, is produced by the pituitary to promote growth in many body cells. To treat children with growth disorders, it has been obtained form primate sources or synthesized. There are reports of abuse by athletes, although there is no clear benefit in taking of the hormone and there are serious side effects, such as acromegaly, from dosages only slightly larger than those given to children.

Hamstrings

The group of muscles at the back of the thigh, and their tendons.

Health history

See medical history.

Health risk appraisal

A procedure that gathers information about a person's behaviors, family history, and other characteristics known to be associated with the incidence of serious disease, and uses that information to compare the individual's present risks with the lower risks that could be achieved by changing certain behaviors.

Heart attack

An acute episode of any kind of heart disease.

Heart rate

Number of heart beats per minute.

Heart rate reserve
The difference between the resting heart rate and the maximal heart rate.

Heat cramps
Muscle twitching or painful cramping, usually following heavy exercise with profuse sweating. The legs, arms, and abdominal muscles are the most often affected.

Heat exhaustion
Caused by dehydration (and sometimes salt loss). Symptoms include dry mouth, excessive thirst, loss of coordination, dizziness, headache, paleness, shakiness, and cool and clammy skin.

Heat stroke
A life threatening illness when the body's temperature-regulating mechanisms fail. Body temperature may rise to over 104 degrees F, skin appears red, dry, and warm to the touch. The victim has chills, sometimes nausea and dizziness, and may be confused or irrational. Seizures and coma may follow unless temperature is brought down to 102 degrees within an hour.

Heat syncope
Fainting from the heat. When a lot of blood is sent to the skin for cooling, and the person becomes inactive enough to allow blood to pool in the legs, the heart may not receive enough blood to supply the brain. Once the person is in a horizontal position, consciousness is regained quickly.

High blood pressure
See hypertension.

High-density lipoprotein (HDL)
A type of lipoprotein that seems to provide protection against the buildup of athersclerotic fat deposits in the arteries. Exercise seems to increase the HDL fraction of total cholesterol. HDL contains high levels of protein and low levels of triglycerides and cholesterol. Cf. lipoprotein, low-density lipoprotein.

Homeostasis
The tendency of the body to maintain its internal systems in balance. Example: A buildup of carbon dioxide increases the respiration rate to eliminate it and draw in more oxygen.

Hormone
A chemical, secreted into the blood stream, that specifically regulates the function of a certain organ of the body. Usually, but not always, secreted by an endocrine gland.

Horsepower
A workrate measure equal to 746 watts, or about 550 foot-pounds per second.

Hyperglycemia
Abnormally high level of glucose in the blood (high blood sugar). The clinical hallmark of diabetes mellitus. Usually defined as a blood sugar value exceeding 140 mg/dl.

Hypertension
Persistent high blood pressure. Readings as low as 140/90 millimeters of mercury are considered a threshold for high blood pressure by some authorities. Cf. blood pressure.

Hyperthermia
Body temperatures exceeding normal. See heat cramps, exhaustion, heat stroke, heat syncope. Cf. hypothermia.

Hypertonic
Describes a solution concentrated enough to draw water out of body cells. Cf. osmolarity.

Hypertrophy
An enlargement of a body part or organ by the increase in size of the cells that make it up. Cf. atrophy.

Hypervitaminosis
Undesirable symptoms caused by an excess of certain vitamins.

Hypoglycemia

Abnormally low level of glucose in the blood (low blood sugar). May lead to shakiness, cold sweats, goose-bumps, hypothermia, hallucinations, strange behavior, and, in extreme cases, convulsions and coma.

Hypothermia

Body temperature below normal. Usually due to exposure to cold temperatures, especially after exhausting ready energy supplies. Cf. hyperthermia.

Hypotonic

Describes a solution dilute enough to allow its water to be absorbed by body cells. Cf. osmolarity.

Hypoxia

Insufficient oxygen flow to the tissues, even though blood flow is adequate. Cf. ischemia.

Iliac crest

The upper, wide portion of the hip bone.

Infarction

Death of a section of tissue from the obstruction of blood flow (ischemia) to the area. Cf. myocardial infarction.

Inflammation

Body's local response to injury. Acute inflammation is characterized by pain, with heat, redness, swelling and loss of function. Uncontrolled swelling may cause further damage to tissues at the injury site.

Informed consent

A procedure for obtaining a client's signed consent to a fitness center's prescription and leadership of his/her program. Includes a description of the objectives and procedures, with associated benefits and risks, stated in plain language, with a consent statement and signature line in a single document.

Inspiration

Breathing air into the lungs. Cf. expiration, respiration.

Intensity

The rate of performing work; power. A function of energy output per unit of time. Examples: Aerobic exercise may be measured in $\dot{V}O_2$, METs, or heart rate; short-duration anaerobic exercise may be measured in foot-pounds per minute or other units of work measurement. Intensity, along with duration and frequency, affect the effectiveness of exercise.

Interval training

An exercise session in which the intensity and duration of exercise are consciously alternated between harder and easier work. Often used to improve aerobic capacity and/or anaerobic endurance in exercisers who already have a base of endurance training.

Ischemia

Inadequate blood flow to a body part, caused by constriction or obstruction of a blood vessel. Cf. hypoxia.

Isokinetic contraction

A muscle contraction against a resistance that moves at a constant velocity, so that the maximum force of which the muscle is capable throughout the range of motion may be applied. Cf. isotonic contraction.

Isometric action

Muscle action in which the muscle attempts to contract against a fixed limit. This is sometimes called "isometric contraction," although there is not appreciable shortening of the muscle.

Isotonic contraction

A muscle contraction against a constant resistance, as in lifting a weight. Cf. isokinetic contraction.

Joint capsules
A sac-like enclosure around a joint that holds synovial fluid to lubricate the joint.

Ketosis
An elevated level of ketone bodies in the tissues. Seen in sufferers of starvation or diabetes, and a symptom brought about in dieters on very low carbohydrate diets.

Kilocalorie (kcal)
A measure of the heat required to raise the temperature of one kilogram of water one degree Celsius. A large Calorie, used in diet and metabolism measures, that equals 1,000 small calories.

Kilogram (kg)
A unit of weight equal to 2.204623 pounds; 1,000 grams (g).

Kilogram-meters (kgm)
The amount of work required to lift one kilogram one meter.

Kilopond-meters (kpm)
Equivalent to kilogram-meters, in normal gravity.

Lactate
Lactic acid.

Lactic acid
The end product of the metabolism of glucose for the anaerobic production of energy.

Lean body mass
Lean body weight.

Lean body weight
The weight of the body, less the weight of its fat.

Ligament
The fibrous, connective tissue that connects bone to bone, or bone to cartilage, to hold together and support joints. Cf. tendon.

Lipid
A number of body substances that are fat or fat-like.

Lipoprotein
Combination of a lipid and protein. Cholesterol is transported in the blood plasma by lipoproteins. Cf. high-density lipoprotein, low-density lipoprotein.

Longitudinal study
A study which observes the same subjects over a period of time. Cf. cross-sectional study.

Lordosis
The forward curving of the spine at the neck (cervical spine) and lower back (lumbar spine). Often used to refer to an abnormally increased curvature of the lumbar spine.

Low blood sugar
See hypoglycemia.

Low-density lipoprotein (LDL)
A lipoprotein carrying a high level of cholesterol, moderate levels of protein and low levels of triglycerides. Associated with the building of athersclerotic deposits in the arteries. Cf. lipoprotein, high-density lipoprotein.

Lumbar
Pertaining to the lower back, defined by the five lumbar vertibrae, just above the sacrum.

Maintenance load
The intensity, duration and frequency of exercise required to maintain an individual's present level of fitness.

Max VO$_2$
See maximal oxygen uptake.

Maximal heart rate
The highest heart rate of which an individual is capable. A broad rule of thumb for

estimating maximal heart rate is 220 (beats per minute) minus the person's age (in years). Cf. graded exercise test.

Maximal oxygen uptake
The highest rate of oxygen consumption of which a person is capable. Usually expressed in milliliters of oxygen per kilogram of body weight per minute. Also called maximal aerobic power, maximal oxygen consumption, maximal oxygen intake. Cf. $\dot{V}O_2$ max.

Maximal tests
An exercise test to exhaustion or to levels of oxygen uptake or heart rate that cannot increase further with additional work loads. Cf. graded exercise test.

Medical history
A list of a person's previous illnesses, present conditions, symptoms, medications and health risk factors. Used to prescribe appropriate exercise programs. Persons whose responses indicate they may be in a high-risk category should be referred for medical evaluation before beginning an exercise program.

Medical referral
Recommending that a person see a qualified medical professional to review their health status and determine whether medical treatment is needed or whether a particular course of exercise and/or diet change is safe.

Met
A measure of energy output equal to the resting metabolic rate of a resting subject. Assumed to be equal to an oxygen uptake of 3.5 milliliters per kilogram of body weight per minute, or a caloric expenditure of 50 Kcalories per square meter of body surface per hour. Hard exercise, for example, requires up to eight METs of energy expenditure, which equals eight times the resting energy requirement.

Metabolism
The total of all the chemical and physical processes by which the body builds and maintains itself (anabolism) and by which it breaks down its substances for the production of energy (catabolism).

Minimum daily requirement (MDR)
The minimum amounts of protein, vitamins and minerals considered necessary to maintain health. Cf. recommended daily allowance.

Monounsaturated fat
Dietary fat whose molecules have one double bond open to receive more hydrogen. Found in many nuts, olive oil, and avocados. Cf. polyunsaturated fat, saturated fat, unsaturated fat.

Motor neuron
A nerve cell which conducts impulses from the central nervous system to a group of muscle fibers to produce movement.

Motor unit
A motor neuron and the muscle fibers activated by it.

Muscle group
Specific muscles that act together at the same joint to produce a movement.

Muscle spindle
Organ in a muscle that senses changes in muscle length, especially stretches. Rapid stretching of the muscle results in messages being sent to the nervous system to contract the muscle, thereby limiting the stretch. Cf. Golgi tendon organ, proprioceptor.

Musculotendinous
Pertaining to or composed of muscle and tendon.

Myocardial infarction
A common form of heart attack, in which the blockage of a coronary artery causes the death of a part of the heart muscle. Cf. infarction.

Myositis
Inflammation of a skeletal muscle.

Myositis ossificans
The deposit of bony materials in the muscle. Bruises from contact sports may result in this condition. Severe bruises should be iced, and evaluated by a physician.

Nutrients
Food and its specific elements and compounds that can be used by the body to build and maintain itself and to produce energy.

Nutrition
The processes involved in taking in and using food substances.

Obesity
Excessive accumulation of body fat.

One repetition maximum (1 RM)
The maximum resistance with which a person can execute one repetition of an exercise movement. Cf. repetition.

Osmolarity
The concentration of a solution participating in osmosis. (E.g., a sugar-water solution of high osmolarity is concentrated enough to draw water through the membranes of the digestive tract to dilute the sugar.) Cf. hypertonic, hypotonic.

Osmosis
The movement of fluid through a membrane, tending to equalize the concentrations of the solutions on both sides. Cf. osmolarity.

Ossification
The formation of bone. The turning of cartilage into bone (as in the joints). Cf. myositis ossificans, osteoarthritis.

Osteoarthritis
A noninflammatory joint disease of older persons. The cartilage in the joint wears down, and there is bone growth at the edges of the joints. Results in pain and stiffness, especially after prolonged exercise. Cf. arthritis.

Overload
Subjecting a part of the body to efforts greater than it is accustomed to, in order to elicit a training response. Increases may be in intensity or duration.

Overuse
Excessive repeated exertion or shock which results in injuries such as stress fractures of bones or inflammation of muscles and tendons.

Oxygen (O$_2$)
The essential element in the respiration process to sustain life. The colorless, odorless gas makes up about 20 percent of the air, by weight at sea level.

Oxygen consumption
See oxygen uptake.

Oxygen debt
The oxygen required to restore the capacity for anaerobic work after an effort has used those reserves. Measured by the extra oxygen that is consumed during the recovery from the work.

Oxygen deficit
The energy supplied anaerobically while oxygen uptake has not yet reached the steady state which matches energy output. Becomes oxygen debt at end of exercise.

Oxygen uptake
The amount of oxygen used up at the cellular level during exercise. Can be measured by determining the amount of oxygen exhaled as compared to the amount inhaled, or estimated by indirect means.

Peak heart rate
The highest heart rate reached during a work session.

APPENDIX
• • •

Perceived exertion

See rating of perceived exertion.

pH

A measure of acidity, relating to the hydrogen ion (H+) concentration. A pH of 7.0 is neutral; acidity increases with lower numbers, and alkalinity increases with higher numbers. Body fluids have a pH of about 7.3.

Physical conditioning

A program of regular, sustained exercise to increase or maintain levels of strength, flexibility, aerobic capacity, and body composition consistent with health, fitness or athletic objectives.

Physical fitness

The physiological contribution to wellness through exercise and nutrition behaviors that maintain high aerobic capacity, balanced body composition, and adequate strength and flexibility to minimize risk of chronic health problems and to enhance the enjoyment of life.

Physical work capacity (PWC)

An exercise test that measures the amount of work done at a given, submaximal heart rate. The work is measured in oxygen uptake, kilopond meters per minute, or other units, and can be used to estimate maximal heart rate and oxygen uptake. Less accurate, but safer and less expensive than the graded exercise test.

Plyometric

A type of exercise that suddenly preloads and forces the stretching of a muscle an instant prior to its concentric action. An example is jumping down from a bench and immediately springing back up.

PNF stretch

See proprioceptive neuromuscular facilitation stretch.

Polyunsaturated fat

Dietary fat whose molecules have more than one double bond open to receive more hydrogen. Found in safflower oil, corn oil, soybeans, sesame seeds, sunflower seeds. Cf. monounsaturated fat, saturated fat, unsaturated fat.

Power

Work performed per unit of time. Measured by the formula: work equals force times distance divided by time. A combination of strength and speed. Cf. strength.

Primary risk factor

A risk factor that is strong enough to operate independently, without the presence of other risk factors. Cf. risk factor, secondary risk factor.

Prime mover

The muscle or muscle group that is causing the movement around a joint. Cf. agonist.

Progressive resistance exercise

Exercise in which the amount of resistance is increased to further stress the muscle after it has become accustomed to handling a lesser resistance.

Pronation

Assuming a face-down position. Of the hand, turning the palm backward or downward. Of the foot, lowering the inner (medial) side of the foot so as to flatten the arch. The opposite of supination.

Proprioceptive neuromuscular facilitation (PNF) stretch

Muscle stretches that use the proprioceptors (muscle spindles) to send inhibiting (relaxing) messages to the muscle that is to be stretched. Example: The contraction of an agonist muscle sends inhibiting signals that relax the antagonist muscle so that it is easier to stretch. (Term was once applied to a very specific therapeutic technique, but now is being widely applied to stretch techniques such as slow-reversal-hold, contract-relax, and hold-relax.)

Proprioceptor
Self-sensors (nerve terminals) that give messages to the nervous system about movements and position of the body. Proprioceptors include muscle spindles and Golgi tendon organs.

Protein
Compounds of amino acids that make up most of the body's cells and perform other physiological functions. Cf. amino acids, essential amino acids.

Pulmonary
Pertaining to the lungs.

Quadriceps
A muscle group at the front of the thigh connected to a common tendon that surrounds the knee cap and attaches to the tibia (lower leg bone). The individual muscles are the rectus femoris, vastus intermedius, vastus lateralis, and vastus medialis. Acts to extend the lower leg.

Radial pulse
The pulse at the wrist.

Rating of perceived exertion
A means to quantify the subjective feeling of the intensity of an exercise. Borg scales, charts which describe a range of intensity from resting to maximal energy outputs, are used as a visual aid to exercisers in keeping their efforts in the effective training zone.

Recommended dietary allowance (RDA)
The protein, vitamin, and mineral amounts considered adequate to meet the nutrition needs of 98 percent of the healthy population. Established by the National Research Council of the National Academy of Sciences. The RDA is calculated to exceed the needs of most people.

Rectus femoris
The long, straight muscle in the front of the thigh which attaches to the knee cap. Part of the quadriceps muscle group.

Rehabilitation
A program to restore physical and psychological independence to persons disabled by illness or injury in the shortest period of time.

Renal
Pertaining to the kidney.

Repetition
An individual completed exercise movement. Repetitions are usually done in multiples. Cf. one repetition maximum, set.

Residual volume
The volume of air remaining in the lungs after a maximum expiration. Must be calculated in the formula for determining body composition through underwater weighing.

Resistance
The force which a muscle is required to work against.

Respiration
Exchange of oxygen and carbon dioxide between the atmosphere and the cells of the body. Includes ventilation (breathing), exchange of gasses to and from the blood in the lungs, transportation of the gasses in the blood, the taking in and utilizing of oxygen, and the elimination of waste products by the cells. Cf. expiration, inspiration, ventilation.

Response
An immediate, short-term change in physiological functions (such as heart-rate or respiration) brought on by exercise. Cf. adaptation.

Retest

A repetition of a given test after passage of time, usually to assess the progress made in an exercise program.

Risk factor

A behavior, characteristic, symptom or sign that is associated with an increased risk of developing a health problem. Example: Smoking is a risk factor for lung cancer and coronary heart disease. Cf. primary risk factor, secondary risk factor.

Saturated fat

Dietary fats whose molecules are saturated with hydrogen. They are usually hard at room temperature and are readily converted into cholesterol in the body. Sources include animal products as well as hydrogenated vegetable oils.

Screening

Comparing individuals to set criteria for inclusion in a fitness program, or for referral to medical evaluation.

Secondary risk factor

A risk factor that acts when certain other risk factors are present. Cf. primary risk factor, risk factor.

Sedentary

Sitting a lot; not involved in any physical activity that might produce significant fitness benefits.

Set

A group of repetitions of an exercise movement done consecutively, without rest, until a given number, or momentary exhaustion, is reached. Cf. repetition.

Shin splints

Pain in the front of the lower leg from inflammation of muscle and tendon tissue caused by overuse. Cf. overuse.

Sign

An indicator of disease found in physician's examination or tests; and objective indicator of disease. Cf. symptom.

Slow-twitch fibers

Muscle fiber type that contracts slowly and is used most in moderate-intensity, endurance exercises, such as distance running. Cf. fast-twitch fibers.

Somatotrophin

See growth hormone.

Spasm

The involuntary contraction of a muscle or muscle group in a sudden, violent manner.

Specificity

The principle that the body adapts very specifically to the training stimuli it is required to deal with. The body will perform best at the specific speed, type of contraction, muscle-group usage, and energy-source usage it has become accustomed to in training.

Spot reducing

An effort to reduce fat at one location on the body by concentrating exercise, manipulation, wraps, etc. on that location. Research indicates that any fat loss is generalized over the body, however.

Sprain

A stretching or tearing of ligaments. Severity ratings of sprains are: first-degree, partial tearing; third-degree, complete tears. Cf. strains.

Static contraction

See isometric action.

Steady state

The physiological stare, during submaximal exercise, where oxygen uptake and heart rate level off, energy demands and energy production are balanced, and the body can maintain the level of exertion for an extended period of time.

Strain

A stretching or tearing of a musculotendinous unit. Degrees of severity include: first-degree, stretching of the unit; second-degree, partial tearing of the unit; third-degree, complete disruption of the unit. Cf. sprain.

Strength

The amount of muscular force that can be exerted. (Speed and distance are not factors of strength.) Cf. power.

Stress

The general physical and psychological response of an individual to any real or perceived adverse stimulus, internal or external, that tends to disturb the individual's homeostasis. Stress that is excessive or reacted to inappropriately, may cause disorders.

Stress fracture

A partial or complete fracture of a bone because of the remodeling process's inability to keep up with the effects of continual, rhythmic, nonviolent stresses on the bone. Cf. overuse.

Stress management

A group of skills for dealing with stresses imposed on an individual without suffering psychological distress and/or physical disorders.

Stress test

See graded exercise test.

Stretching

Lengthening a muscle to its maximum extension; moving a joint to the limits of its extension.

Stroke volume

The volume of blood pumped out of the heart by the ventricles in one contraction.

Submaximal

Less than maximum. Submaximal exercise requires less than one's maximum oxygen uptake, heart rate, or anaerobic power. Usually refers to intensity of the exercise, but may be used to refer to duration.

Supination

Assuming a horizontal position facing upward. In the case of the hand, it also means turning the palm to face forward. The opposite of pronation.

Symptom

Any evidence by which a person perceives that he/she may not be well; subjective evidence of illness. Cf. sign.

Syncope

Fainting. A temporary loss of consciousness from insufficient blood flow to the brain.

Syndrome

A group of related symptoms or signs of disease.

Systole

The contraction, or time of contraction, of the heart. Cf. diastole.

Systolic blood pressure

Blood pressure during the contraction of the heart muscle. Cf. blood pressure.

Tachycardia

Excessively rapid heart rate. Usually describes a pulse of more than 100 beats per minute at rest. Cf. bradycardia.

Taper down

See cool down.

Target heart rate (THR)

The heart rate at which one aims to exercise at a THR of 60 to 90 percent of maximum heart rate reserve.

Tendon
The fibrous connective tissue that connects muscle to bone. Cf. ligament.

Tendonitis
Inflammation of a tendon.

Testing protocol
A specific plan for the conducting of a testing situation; usually following an accepted standard.

Testosterone
The sex hormone that predominates in the male, is responsible for the development of male secondary sex characteristics and is involved in the hypertrophy of muscle. Cf. estrogen.

Training
Subjecting the body to repeated stresses with interspersed recovery periods to elicit growth in its capacity to handle such stresses.

Training zone
See target heart rate.

Twitch
A brief muscle contraction caused by a single volley of motor neuron impulses. Cf. fast-twitch fibers, slow-twitch fibers.

Unsaturated fat
Dietary fat whose molecules have one or more double bonds to receive more hydrogen atoms. Replacing saturated fats with unsaturated fats in the diet can help reduce cholesterol levels. Cf. monounsaturated fat, polyunsaturated fat, saturated fat.

Valsalva maneuver
A strong exhaling effort against a closed glottis, which builds pressure in the chest cavity that interferes with the return of the blood tho the heart. May deprive the brain of blood and cause fainting.

Vasoconstriction
The narrowing of a blood vessel to decrease blood flow to a body part.

Vasodilation
The enlarging of a blood vessel to increase blood flow to a body part.

Vein
A vessel which returns blood from the various parts of the body back to the heart.

Ventilation
Breathing. Cf. expiration, inspiration, respiration.

Vertigo
Sensation that the world is spinning or that the individual is revolving; a particular kind of dizziness.

Vital capacity
Maximal breathing capacity; the amount of air that can be expired after a maximum inspiration; the maximum total volume of the lungs, less the residual volume.

Vital signs
The measurable signs of essential bodily functions, such as respiration rate, heart rate, temperature, blood pressure, etc.

Vitamins
A number of unrelated organic substances that are required in trace amounts for the metabolic processes of the body, and which occur in small amounts in many foods.

$\dot{V}O_2$ max
Maximum volume of oxygen consumed per unit of time. In scientific notation, a dot appears over the V to indicate "per unit of time." Cf. maximal oxygen uptake.

Warm-up

A gradual increase in the intensity of exercise to allow physiological processes to prepare for greater energy outputs. Changes include: rise in body temperature, cardiovascular- and respiratory-system changes, increase in muscle elasticity and contractility, etc.

Watt

A measure of power equal to 6.12 kilogram-meters per minute.

Wellness

A state of health more positive than the mere absence of disease. Wellness programs emphasize self-responsibility for a lifestyle process that realizes the individual's highest physical, mental, and spiritual well-being.

Wet-bulb thermometer

A thermometer whose bulb is enclosed in a wet wick, so that evaporation from the wick will lower the temperature reading more in dry air than in humid air. The comparison of wet-and dry-bulb readings can be used to calculate relative humidity. Cf. dry-bulb thermometer, wet-globe temperature.

Wet-globe temperature

A temperature reading that approximates the heat stress which the environment will impose on the human body. Takes into account not only temperature and humidity, but radiant heat from the sun and cooling breezes that would speed evaporation and convection of heat away from the body. Reading is provided by an instrument that encloses a thermometer in a wetted, black copper sphere. Cf. dry-bulb thermometer, wet-bulb thermometer.

Work

Force times distance. Measured in foot-pounds and similar units. Example: Lifting a 200-pound barbell 8 feet and lifting a 400-pound barbell 4 feet each require 1,600 foot-pounds of work.

Work measures

See foot-pounds, kilogram-meters.

Workout

A complete exercise session, ideally consisting of warm-up, intense aerobic and/or strength exercises, and cool-down.

Workrate

Power. The amount of work done per unit of time. Can be measured in foot-pounds per second, watts, horsepower, etc.

APPENDIX B

GUIDELINES FOR PERFORMING CPR

GUIDELINES FOR PERFORMING CPR

Being trained in the basic life support (BLS) methods of cardiopulmonary resuscitation (CPR) is essential for individuals who supervise exercise tests and training programs, and strongly recommended for everyone. The major objective of CPR is to promote the oxygenation of the brain, heart, and other vital organs.

The acronym for remembering the techniques of CPR is *ABC*—Airway, Breathing and Circulation. An initial assessment to determine responsiveness breathing and circulation (i.e., the presence of a pulse) is required before starting CPR. This assessment should take only a few seconds. The recommended techniques for CPR performed by one person (i.e., one-rescuer*) involve the following steps:

- *Airway.* Tap, gently shake, and shout at the victim; call for help; position the victim supine (on his/her back, face up) on a firm surface; open the airway by lightly pressing down on the victim's forehead with one hand while gently lifting their chin with your other hand (i.e., the head-tilt/chin-lift maneuver); clear the victim's mouth of any visible obstruction.
- *Breathing.* Look, listen, and feel for signs of breathing by the victim (3-5 seconds); give the victim two full breaths.
- *Circulation.* Feel the carotid artery (located near the Adam's apple). If no pulse is detected, perform 15 external chest compressions at a rate of 80-100 per minute; count aloud "one," "two," and so on to "fifteen"; open the airway (tilt) and give two full breaths as before; repeat the 15 chest compressions; perform four complete cycles of 15 compressions and two ventilations.
- *Reassessment.* After completing the four cycles (15:2 ratio— compression:ventilations), reevaluate the victim. Check the carotid pulse for 5-10 seconds; if no pulse is detected, resume CPR starting with two full breaths. Check again for breathing. The CPR procedure should not be stopped until appropriate medical help arrives.

All exercise personnel should be trained in both the one- and two-rescuer CPR techniques. A compression rate of 80-100 per minute should be employed for both techniques. Unlike the one-rescuer CPR method, the two-rescuer approach involves a compression:ventilation ratio of 5:1, with a 1-1.5 second pause for ventilation. Prompt action is the key to successful CPR regardless of which method you use.

---

*If someone other than the rescuer is present, have that person immediately call the EMS (emergency medical services - 911). If you are alone, perform CPR for one minute, then call the EMS.

APPENDIX C

GUIDELINES FOR EXERCISING ON THE STAIRMASTER® EXERCISE SYSTEMS

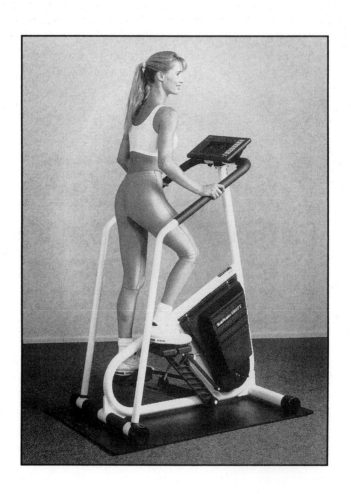

APPENDIX C-1

• •

HOW TO PROPERLY USE
THE STAIRMASTER® 4000PT®*

The StairMaster 4000PT has an independent stepping action that enables you to achieve effective aerobic and lower body conditioning with little or no orthopaedic trauma. You can derive the most benefits from your stair climbing efforts by adhering to the following guidelines:

- Select a stepping rate (i.e., exercise intensity) that allows you to stay in the middle of the range of motion for the pedals. The key is to select a climbing speed which enables you to achieve a training effect and enjoy the activity. Faster is not always better. Work out at a level that is consistent with your functional capabilities, needs, and interests. (Note: One easy method for increasing the difficulty of your workout is to refrain from using the handrails—even for balance—while exercising.)
- Exercise for approximately 15-20 minutes. If necessary, take a brief rest period while you're exercising, but make sure that you exercise collectively for a minimum of 15-20 minutes. Once you improve your fitness level and become more comfortable on the machine, gradually extend the amount of time you exercise to 30 minutes or more (Note: It is generally recommended that individuals not exceed 60 minutes of exercise on the StairMaster 4000PT at any one time in order to reduce the likelihood of overtraining.)
- Don't let the pedals (steps) contact either the floor or the upper stop levels. Such contact, not only can cause trauma to your joints, but can result in a jerky, uncomfortable motion.
- Don't lean on the console or the handrails of the machine. Partially supporting yourself on the machine will decrease the work level at which you're exercising (by lowering the amount of weight you have to lift during each step), thereby decreasing the number of calories actually expend during the exercise bout. Leaning forward on a machine while exercising can also put your back in a possibly injurious (flexed) position.
- Relax as much as possible while stair climbing and maintain an erect posture. If possible, let your arms hang naturally.

These guidelines also apply to the StairMaster® 4000CT™.

• • •

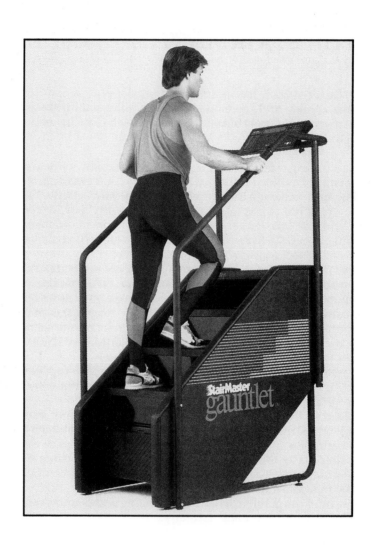

HOW TO PROPERLY USE THE
STAIRMASTER® GAUNTLET®

The StairMaster Gauntlet is a vertical treadmill-like device which has a revolving staircase that allows you to experience the proven training benefits of conventional stair climbing without the orthopaedic trauma. To gain the most from exercising on the Gauntlet, you should adhere to the following guidelines:

- Select a stepping rate (i.e., exercise intensity) that allows you to stay in the middle of the staircase. The key is to select a climbing speed which enables you to achieve a training effect and enjoy the activity. Faster is not always better. Work out at a level that is consistent with your functional capabilities, needs, and interests. (Note: One effective method for increasing the difficulty of your workout is to refrain from using the handrails—even for balance—while exercising.)
- Exercise for approximately 15-20 minutes. Take a brief rest period if you have to while you're exercising, but make sure that you exercise collectively for a minimum of 15-20 minutes. Once you improve your fitness level and become more comfortable on the machine, gradually extend the amount of time you exercise to 30 minutes or more (Note: It is generally recommended that individuals not exceed 60 minutes of exercise on the Gauntlet at any one time in order to reduce the likelihood of overtraining.)
- Don't lean on the console or the handrails of the machine. Partially supporting yourself on the machine will decrease the work level at which you're exercising (by lowering the amount of weight you have to lift during each step), thereby decreasing the number of calories you actually expend during the exercise bout. Leaning forward on a machine while exercising can also put your back in a possibly injurious (flexed) position.
- Relax as much as possible while stair climbing and maintain an erect posture. If possible, let your arms hang naturally.

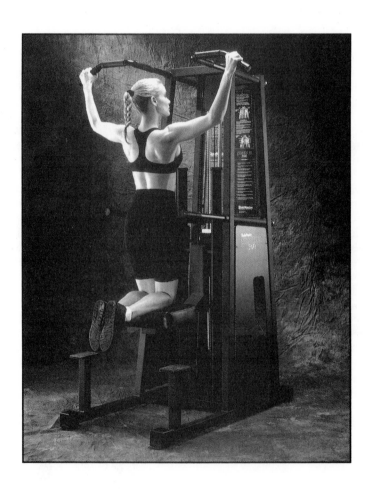

• •

HOW TO PROPERLY USE THE
STAIRMASTER® GRAVITRON 2000™

The StairMaster Gravitron 2000 features a weight stack user-assistance mechanism which enables you to properly perform bar dips, pull-ups, and chin-ups at a level of resistance that you can handle. The following guidelines provide the basic information and instruction that you need to safely and effectively use the Gravitron 2000:

- Mount the Gravitron 2000 by using the assistance steps. Assume a kneeling position on the support platform. Maintain an erect body position on the platform while exercising.
- Perform bar dips by assuming a starting position with your arms fully extended on the dip bars. Start the exercise by lowering your body by bending your arms until your upper arms are approximately parallel to the dip bars. Recover to the starting position by extending your arms.
- Perform pull-ups or chin-ups by assuming a starting position by hanging from the overhead bar with your arms fully extended. Slowly pull upward until your chin is above the level of your hands. Recover to the starting position by slowly lowering your body.
- Perform three sets of both dips and pull-ups (or chin-ups) each workout. Each set should consist of a minimum of ten repetitions of the exercise. Alternate one set of dips with one set of pull-ups (or chin-ups) and so on until your workout is completed.
- Dismount by stepping onto the assistance steps and allowing the weight stack to slowly return to its resting position.

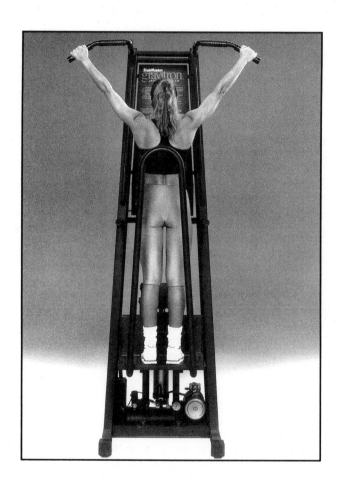

APPENDIX C-4

HOW TO PROPERLY USE THE STAIRMASTER® GRAVITRON®

The StairMaster Gravitron features a pneumatically (air) powered platform that provides lift assistance which is designed to enable you to properly perform bar dips, pull-ups and chin-ups at a level of resistance that you can handle. The following guidelines provide the basic information and instruction that you need to safely and effectively use the Gravitron:

- Step onto the platform and stand erect.
- Press the large red ON/OFF switch at the right side on the computer console.
- Enter your (accurate) body weight (in pounds or, if you have a metric console, in kilograms) on the key pad and press the ENT (enter) key. Entry errors may be erased simply by pressing the CLR (clear) key.
- Select the difficulty level at which you would like to exercise (difficulty level #1 or 10% of your body weight to difficulty level #17 or 90% of your body weight) and press ENT.
- Wait until the air compressor stops running and the pace light in the LEVEL/ PACE window moves up and down to display a suggested pace. (Note: If you attempt to do a dip, pull-up, or chin-up while the air compressor is running, the compressor will automatically stop and the system will depressurize.)
- Start exercising with your hands on the dip bars. Push your body upward until your arms are fully extended. Then lower your body by bending your elbows until your upper arms are approximately parallel to the dip bars. Remain erect throughout the exercise movement. As much as possible, exercise at a speed which follows the pace light. (Note: To receive lift assistance, you must remain in contact with the platform at all times).
- After you have performed a set of ten repetitions of the dip exercise, reach up and grasp the overhead bar at any one of the three grip positions (parallel, military, or wide) so that you can perform chin-ups or pull-ups (if necessary, you may step up on the step pad in front of the platform so that you can reach the pull-up bar). Slowly pull your body upward until your chin is above the level of your hands; then slowly lower your body until your arms are extended. Follow the pace light. Perform ten repetitions.
- Repeat until you have alternately performed three sets each of dips and pull-ups/ chin-ups.

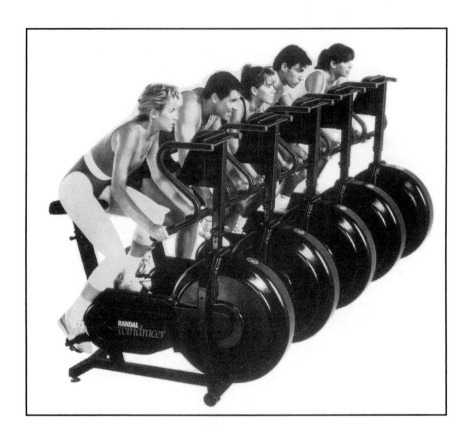

APPENDIX D

• •

GUIDELINES FOR EXERCISING ON THE WINDRACER® EXERCISE SYSTEMS

• •

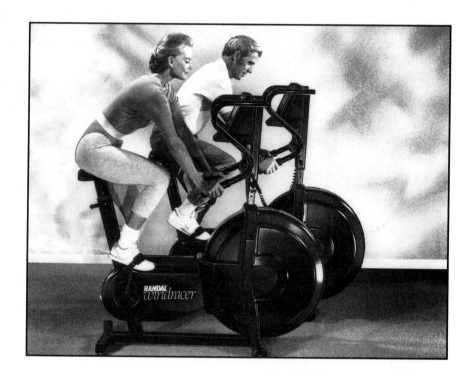

APPENDIX D-1

●●

HOW TO PROPERLY USE THE WINDRACER™ CYCLE

Cycling is an excellent form of aerobic exercise that places a substantial demand on your heart and lungs. All factors considered, it is a very safe form of exercise since it imposes far less stress on the joints of your body than many other types of aerobic exercise. When you exercise on the Windracer exercise cycle, you should adhere to the following basic guidelines to ensure that your efforts are safe, effective, and enjoyable:

- Adjust the seat and handlebars to a position that is comfortable for you. For most individuals, the seat and handlebars are in an appropriate setting when they are placed at the same positioning number (#1-#6).
- Position the seat so that at the bottom of the stroke your knee is slightly bent when the ball of your foot is on the pedal. A quick guide for determining if your seat height is too high for you is to try backpedalling—if you are required to rock your hips or if your heels slip off the pedals, your seat is too high.
- Pedal in a circular motion, pulling up with one foot while pushing down with the other one. This technique is more efficient than simply pushing only on the downstroke. Be sure to also drop your heel at the bottom of the stroke, and raise it at the top; this action will ensure that any forces on your knee joint are safely distributed.
- Exercise for at least 15-20 minutes at a level of intensity that is sufficient to produce a training effect.

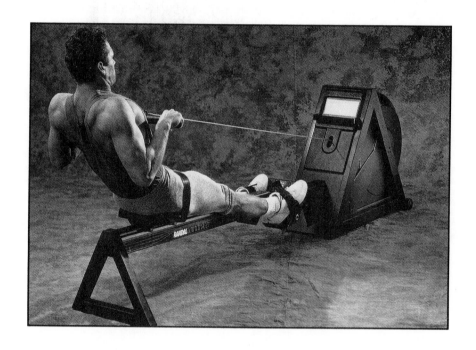

APPENDIX D-2

• •

HOW TO PROPERLY USE THE WINDRACER™ ROWER

As a means for developing aerobic fitness, rowing can be an excellent modality. Not only do rowing machines enable you to develop your cardiorespiratory system, they also place a considerable demand on your muscular system—particularly of the upper body. In general, you should adhere to the following basic guidelines and techniques when using the Windracer rower:

- Select an exercise program and intensity level, and input required information into the computer console.
- Place your feet on the platform and secure the foot straps. Leave the foot straps sufficiently loose so that you can lift your heels when you slide forward at the beginning of the stroke.
- Begin the rowing stroke with your arms extended.
- Push with your legs; keep your arms straight.
- Complete the stroke by pulling the handle into your abdomen; extend your legs.
- Recover to the starting position by first extending your arms and then bending your legs.
- Exercise for at least 15-20 minutes at a level of intensity that is sufficient to produce a training effect.

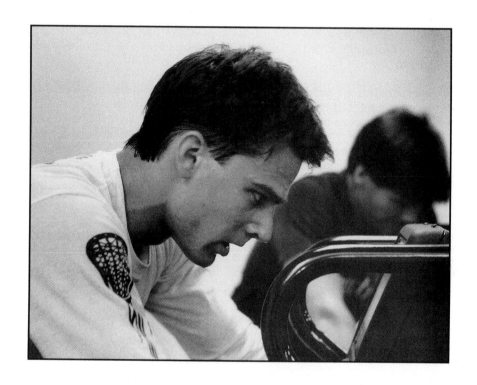

Appendix E

SIGNS OR SYMPTOMS OF OVERTRAINING

SIGNS OR SYMPTOMS
OF OVERTRAINING

Part of the "art" of prescribing exercise is the ability to design your program in such a manner that it provides a sufficient training stimulus to induce positive physiological changes without exceeding your body's adaptive capabilities. Overtraining is a term that is used to express the situation when an imbalance (as described above) occurs between training and recovery. The symptoms of overtraining can vary from one individual to another. The most common signs or symptoms of overtraining , however, frequently involve one or more of the following:

- impaired physical performance
- reduced enthusiasm and desire for training
- increased resting heart rate (i.e., your heart rate taken first thing in the morning— before arising out of bed)
- increased resting blood pressure
- chronic muscle or joint soreness
- increased incidence of musculoskeletal injuries
- increased incidence of colds and infections
- impaired recovery from exercise (e.g., heart rate remains elevated well after the completion of a bout of exercise)
- increased perceived exertion during your normal workouts
- reduced appetite
- weight loss
- disturbed sleep patterns
- increased depression, irritability, or anxiety

Appendix F

SAMPLE EXERCISE RECORDING FORMS

SAMPLE AEROBIC EXERCISE RECORDING FORM

Name_____

Month_____

Date	Body* Weight	Type of Exercise	Distance In Miles	Time In Mins.	Exercise Heart Rate	Recovery# Heart Rate	RPE†	Enjoyment Level§
1								
2								
3								
4								
5								
6								
7								
8								
9								
10								
11								
12								
13								
14								
15								
16								
17								
18								
19								
20								
21								
22								
23								
24								
25								
26								
27								
28								
29								
30								
31								

* Body weight should not be recorded more frequently than once per week
\# Heart rate taken two minutes post-exercise
\+ Rating of perceived exertion
§ How enjoyable was the exercise bout (1=the lowest level of enjoyment and 5=the highest level of enjoyment)?

SAMPLE STRENGTH TRAINING RECORDING FORM

Name_____

Date					
Body Weight*					
Enjoyment Level§					
Exercise	St/Reps/Res#	St/Reps/Res	St/Reps/Res	St/Reps/Res	St/Reps/Res

* Body weight should not be recorded more frequently than once per week
§ How enjoyable was the exercise bout (1=the lowest level of enjoyment and 5=the highest level of enjoyment)?
# St/Reps/Res = Sets, Repetitions, and Resistence (e.g., 1/10/135 = 1 set of 10 repetitions with 135 pounds)

SAMPLE FLEXIBILITY TRAINING RECORDING FORM

Name_____

Date				
Exercise	Reps*/Time§/Type#	Reps*/Time§/Type#	Reps*/Time§/Type#	Reps*/Time§/Type#

* The number of times a given stretching exercise is performed
§ The duration that each stretch is held. In general, 10-30 seconds is the recommended length of time that each stretch should be held
# Stretching can be performed in several ways, static stretching (i.e., slowly stretching a muscle past its normal length and holding the stretch) is considered to be the safest manner in which to stretch

APPENDIX G

SELECTING EXERCISES
TO DEVELOP
MUSCULAR FITNESS

SELECTING EXERCISES TO DEVELOP MUSCULAR FITNESS

Considerable latitude exists concerning how you organize your developmental program for muscular fitness. Based on existing research and empirical evidence, the following basic guidelines can be used identify which exercises should be incorporated into your strength training program:

1. As a general rule, at the minimum, your strength training program should include exercises for each of the major muscle areas in your body:
   • Lower back and buttocks
   • Legs
   • Torso
   • Arms
   • Abdominals

2. The selection of what specific exercises you should perform to develop a particular muscle area should be based on at least three factors:
   • Personal preference
   • Availability of equipment
   • Safety

   Figure G-1 illustrates the muscles of the body and lists several of the more commonly performed exercises for those muscles. Table G-1 provides an overview of possible exercises using different kinds of equipment for selected muscles of the body.

3. Whenever possible, exercises which involve pushing movements should be alternated with exercises which involve pulling movements. Table G-2 lists four sample strength workouts which include 12 exercises each. Depending upon your interests and needs, the final "recipe" of exercises is often a matter of personal preference.

Figure G-1. Commonly Performed Exercises for the Major Muscle Areas of the Body.

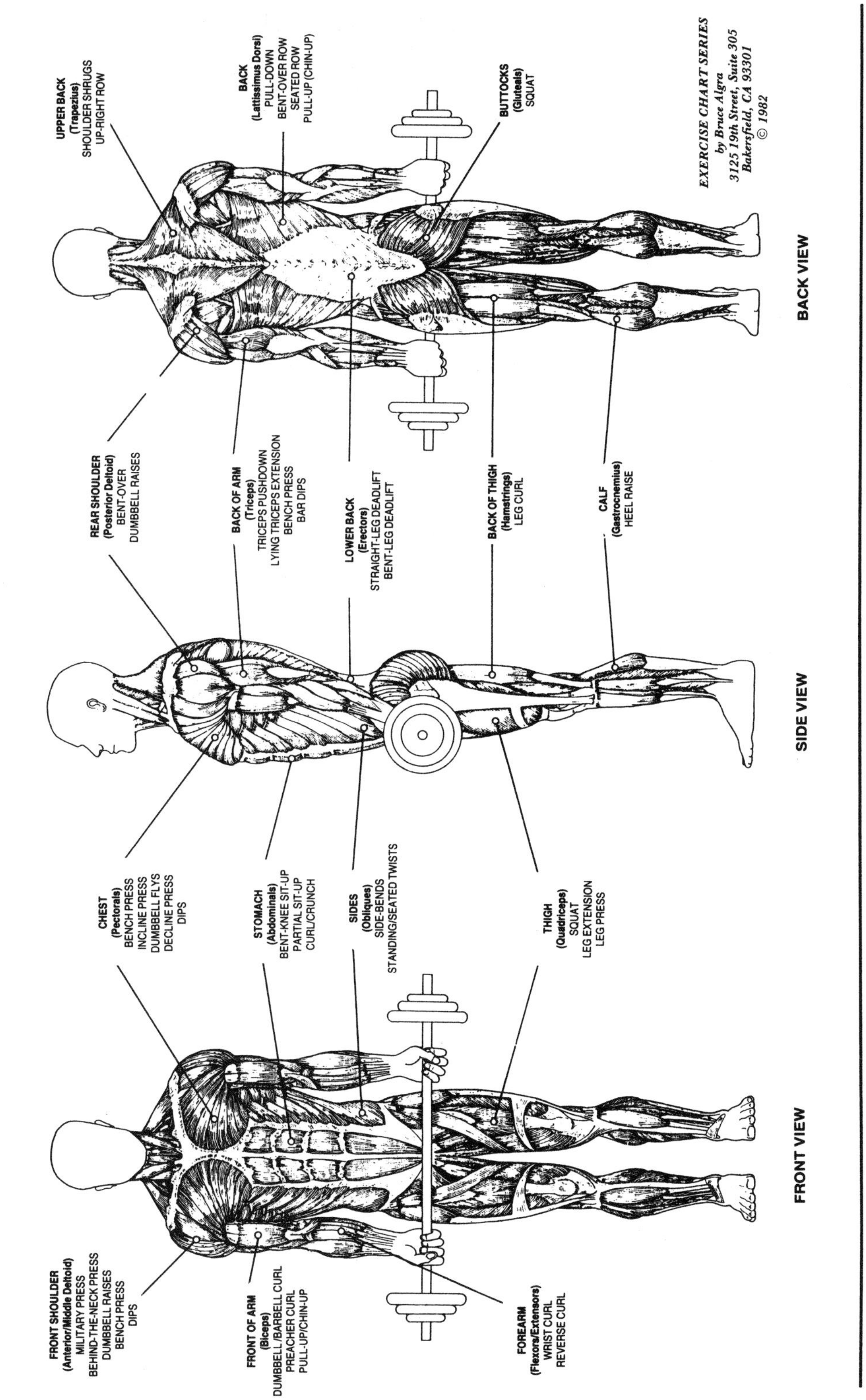

FRONT SHOULDER
(Anterior/Middle Deltoid)
MILITARY PRESS
BEHIND-THE-NECK PRESS
DUMBBELL RAISES
BENCH PRESS
DIPS

FRONT OF ARM
(Biceps)
DUMBBELL/BARBELL CURL
PREACHER CURL
PULL-UP/CHIN-UP

FOREARM
(Flexors/Extensors)
WRIST CURL
REVERSE CURL

CHEST
(Pectorals)
BENCH PRESS
INCLINE PRESS
DUMBBELL FLYS
DECLINE PRESS
DIPS

STOMACH
(Abdominals)
BENT-KNEE SIT-UP
PARTIAL SIT-UP
CURL/CRUNCH

SIDES
(Obliques)
SIDE-BENDS
STANDING/SEATED TWISTS

THIGH
(Quadriceps)
SQUAT
LEG EXTENSION
LEG PRESS

REAR SHOULDER
(Posterior Deltoid)
BENT-OVER
DUMBBELL RAISES

BACK OF ARM
(Triceps)
TRICEPS PUSHDOWN
LYING TRICEPS EXTENSION
BENCH PRESS
BAR DIPS

LOWER BACK
(Erectors)
STRAIGHT-LEG DEADLIFT
BENT-LEG DEADLIFT

BACK OF THIGH
(Hamstrings)
LEG CURL

CALF
(Gastrocnemius)
HEEL RAISE

UPPER BACK
(Trapezius)
SHOULDER SHRUGS
UP-RIGHT ROW

BACK
(Lattissimus Dorsi)
PULL-DOWN
BENT-OVER ROW
SEATED ROW
PULL-UP (CHIN-UP)

BUTTOCKS
(Gluteals)
SQUAT

FRONT VIEW

SIDE VIEW

BACK VIEW

EXERCISE CHART SERIES
by Bruce Algra
3125 19th Street, Suite 305
Bakersfield, CA 93301
© 1982

Table G-1. Strength Training Exercises for Selected Muscles.

LOWER BODY MUSCLES	EXERCISES			
	FREE WEIGHTS	MULTI-STATION GYM	VARIABLE RESISTANCE MACHINES	BUDDY EXERCISES

ERECTOR SPINAE	Squat
	Bent-legged
	  Dead Lift
	Straight-legged
	  Dead Lift
		Back Extension	Hip Extension	Squat
				Back Extension

BUTTOCKS	Squat
	Bent-legged
	  Dead Lift
	Leg Press (AMF)
	Step Up
	Straight-legged
	  Dead Lift
		Leg Press	Hip Extension
			Leg Press
			Hip Abduction
				Squat
				Leg Press
				Hip Abduction

QUADRICEPS	Squat Bent-legged Dead Lift Leg Press (AMF) Step Up	Leg Extension Leg Press	Leg Extension Leg Press Hip Abduction	Leg Press Leg Extension
HAMSTRINGS	Squat Bent-legged Dead Lift Leg Press (AMF)		Leg Curl	Leg Curl Squat
HIP FLEXORS	Step Up			Hip Flexion
HIP EXTENSIORS	Squat			
CALVES	Heel Raise	Heel Raise	Heel Raise	Heel Raise
ADDUCTOR MAGNUS			Hip Adduction	Hip Adduction

UPPER BODY MUSCLES*	EXERCISES			
	FREE WEIGHTS	MULTI-STATION GYM	VARIABLE RESISTANCE MACHINES	BUDDY EXERCISES

DELTOIDS	Upright Row
	Bench Press
		Upright Row
		Bench Press
			Arm Cross
			Rowing Torso
			Seated Press
				Bench Press
				Bent-Arm Fly
				Front Raise
				Bent-over Side
				  Lateral Raise
				Seated Press
				Supine
				  Pulldown

TRAPEZIUS	Upright Row
	Shoulder Shrug
		Upright Row
		Shoulder Shrug
			Shoulder Shrug	Shoulder Shrug
				Bent-over Side
				  Lateral Raise
				Supine
				  Pulldown

ROTATOR CUFF	Internal
	  Rotation
	External
	  Rotation
				Internal
				  Rotation
				External
				  Rotation

RHOMBOIDS	Bent-over Fly		Rowing Torso	Back Pulldown Bent-over Side Lateral Raise

LATISSIMUS DORSI	Pull-up/Chin-up
	Bent-over Row
	Bent-over Fly
		Lat Pulldown
		Pull-up/
		  Chin-up
			Pull-up/
			  Chin-up
			Pullover
				Lat Pulldown

PECTORALS	Bench Press	Bench Press	Arm Cross	Bench Press Bent-arm Fly Front Raise
BICEPS	Pull-up/Chin-up Bent-over Row Bicep Curl	Upright Row Bicep Curl Lat Pulldown Pull-up/Chin-up	Pull-up/ Chin-up Two-arm Curl	Bicep Curl Lat Pulldown Back Pulldown
TRICEPS	French Curl Bench Press Dips	Tricep Extension Bench Press Dips	Tricep Extension	Tricep Extension Bench Press Seated Press

FOREARM EXTENSORS/ FLEXORS	Wrist Curl
	Reverse
	  Wrist Curl
		Wrist Curl
		Reverse
		  Wrist Curl
			Wrist Curl
			Reverse
			  Wrist Curl	

* We recommend that you perform abdominal curls/crunches or bent-knee partial sit-ups for training your abdominal region.

Table G-2.   Sample Strength Training Workouts.

FREE WEIGHT WORKOUT

- Squat
- Step-up
- Heel Raise
- Bench Press
- Bent-over Ros
- Upright Row
- Shoulder Shrug
- Pull-ups/Chin-ups
- Dips
- Abdominal Curl

MULTI-STATION MACHINE WORKOUT

- Leg Press
- Leg Extension
- Leg Curl
- Heel Raise
- Bench Press
- Lat Pulldown
- Seated Press
- Pull-ups/Chin-ups
- Dips
- Abdominal Curl

VARIABLE RESISTANCE MACHINE WORKOUT

- Leg Press
- Leg Extension
- Leg Curl
- Heel Raise
- Pectoral Fly
- Pullover
- Seated Press
- Pull-ups/Chin-ups
- Dips
- Abdominal Curl

BUDDY EXERCISE WORKOUT

- Leg Press
- Leg Extension
- Leg Curl
- Heel Raise
- Push-up
- Seated Row
- Seated Press
- Biceps Curl
- Triceps Extension
- Abdominal Curl

*   Your workout should consist of 8-10 exercises for the major muscle groups (areas) and 2-4 exercises for the accessory muscle groups. selecting a modality to develop aerobic fitness

APPENDIX H

SELECTING A MODALITY
TO DEVELOP
AEROBIC FITNESS

SELECTING A MODALITY TO DEVELOP AEROBIC FITNESS

Considerable latitude exists concerning what means you use to develop aerobic fitness. Based on existing research and empirical evidence, the following basic guidelines can be employed to identify which modality would be appropriate for your aerobic fitness program:

1. As a general rule, the modality you use to develop your level of aerobic fitness should have the following features:

    • Involve the large muscles in your body
    • Be rhythmic in nature
    • Can be performed in a continuous, sustained fashion

2. The selection of what specific modality you should use to develop aerobic fitness should be based on at least four factors:

    • Your existing level of fitness
    • Personal preference
    • Availability of equipment
    • Safety

3. Whenever possible, if you perform aerobic activities which are relatively high in the degree of orthopaedic impact to which they subject you, you should alternate those activities with types of aerobic exercise which have either no impact or low impact. Table H-1 offers a comparative overview of the relative advantages and disadvantages of the most popular aerobic modalities. Depending upon your interests and needs, the final "choice" of aerobic modality is primarily a matter of personal preference.

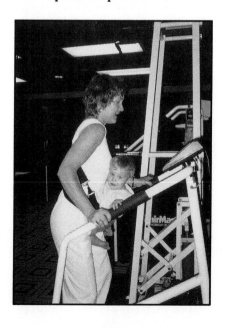

Table H-1. A Comparative Overview of Selected Aerobic Modalities.

	Orthopaedic Impact	Cost *	Skill Involved	Weight Bearing **	Environmental Limitation
Walking	Minimal	Low	Low	Yes	Possible
Jogging	High	Low	Low	Yes	Possible
Stair Climbing (Independent)	None	High	Low	Yes	No
Stair Climbing (Dependent)	High	High	Low	Yes	No
Exercise Cycling	None	High	Low	No	No
Swimming	None	Low	High	No	Possible
Treadmill	Moderate	High	Low	Yes	No
Bicycling	None	Moderate	Low	No	Possible
Rowing (Indoors)	None	High	Low	No	No
Cross Country Skiing (Indoors)	None	Moderate	High	Yes	No

*   The costs are relative. If you have to join a facility to swim, for example, the expense can be somewhat high. By the same token, if you spend a lot on running gear (shoes, outfit, etc.), the costs can easily mount.

**   A growing body of evidence suggests that weight-bearing exercise plays an extremely important role in the maintenance of proper bone health.

STAIRMASTER® SPORTS/MEDICAL PRODUCTS, INC.: OFFICES IN THE UNITED STATES

CORPORATE HEADQUARTERS
12421 Willows Road NE, Suite 100
Kirkland, WA 98034
(800) 635-2936
(206) 823-1825
Customer Service FAX (206) 820-8666

MANUFACTURING DIVISION
6015 North Xanthus
Tulsa, OK 74130
(800) 331-3578
(918) 425-5588
Customer Service FAX (918) 425-4852

EAST REGION
(800) 772-0089
(914) 564-6011
FAX (914) 564-8157
Serving: Connecticut, New Jersey,
          New York, Pennsylvania

NEW ENGLAND AREA
(800) 772-0089
(617) 229-0045
FAX (617) 229-0357
Serving: Maine, Massachusetts, New
          Hampshire, Rhode Island, Vermont

SOUTHEAST REGION
(800) 448-5040
(813) 531-5040
FAX (813) 539-1342
Serving: Alabama, Florida, Georgia,
          Mississippi, North Carolina
          South Carolina

MID-ATLANTIC AREA
(800) 448-5043
(703) 803-9650
FAX (703) 803-9522
Serving: Delaware, Maryland, Virginia,
          Washington, D.C.

WEST REGION
(800) 829-9993
(805) 495-6414
FAX (805) 498-2314
Serving: Arizona, California, Colorado,
          Hawaii, Nevada, New Mexico, Utah

BAY AREA
(800) 829-9993
(510) 463-1181
FAX (510) 463-1636
Serving: Northern California and
          Northern Nevada

NORTHWEST AREA
(800) 733-3783
(206) 820-7764
FAX (206) 820-7505
Serving: Alaska, Idaho, Montana,
          Oregon, Washington, Wyoming

SOUTHWEST REGION
(800) 777-4348
(918) 493-2099
FAX (918) 494-6661
Serving: Arkansas, Kansas, Louisiana,
          Missouri, Nebraska, North Dakota,
          Oklahoma, South Dakota, Texas

MID-AMERICA REGION
(800) 950-2814
(216) 425-4833
FAX (216) 425-4829
Serving: Kentucky, Michigan, Ohio,
          Tennessee, West Virginia

MIDWEST AREA
(800) 800-0957
(708) 231-5010
FAX (708) 231-9197
Serving: Illinois, Indiana, Iowa,
          Minnesota, Wisconsin

STAIRMASTER® SPORTS/MEDICAL PRODUCTS, INC.: INTERNATIONAL OFFICES

INTERNATIONAL DIVISION
(800) 635-2936
(206) 823-1825
FAX (206) 820-7505

GERMANY: HEADQUARTERS
49-2204/610-27
FAX 49-2204/219-66

AUSTRALIA: HEADQUARTERS
61-3/800-2122
FAX 61-3/800-2722

EUROPE: HEADQUARTERS
49-2204/610-27
FAX 49-2204/219-66

CANADA: HEADQUARTERS
(800) 668-4857
(416) 798-2670
FAX (416) 798-2679

JAPAN: HEADQUARTERS
81-03-5479-6711
FAX 81-03-5479-6711

UNITED KINGDOM: HEADQUARTERS
44-908/221-323
FAX 44-908/223-162

COUNTRIES NOT LISTED
(800) 635-2936
FAX (206) 820-7505

ABOUT THE EDITORS

JAMES A. PETERSON, PH.D. is the Director of Sports Medicine for StairMaster Sports/Medical Products, Inc. Dr. Peterson was formerly a professor in the Department of Physical Education at the United States Military Academy in West Point, New York. He is an accomplished author with over thirty published books on exercise, fitness and health.

CEDRIC X. BRYANT, PH.D. is the Associate Director of Sports Medicine for StairMaster Sports/Medical Products, Inc. Prior to assuming his present position, he served on the Exercise Science and Physical Education faculties of the United States Military Academy at West Point, Penn State University and Arizona State University. He is certified as an exercise specialist by the American College of Sports Medicine.